HEAVY *Snow*

My Father's Disappearance into Alzheimer's

John Haugse

Health Communications, Inc.
Deerfield Beach, Florida

www.hci-online.com

Library of Congress Cataloging-in-Publication Data

Haugse, John E.
    Heavy snow: my father's disappearance into Alzheimer's / John Haugse.
      p.   cm.
    ISBN 1-55874-677-3 (trade paper)
    1. Alzheimer's disease Miscellanea.   I. Title.
RC523.2.H38   1999
362.1'96831—dc21

          99-34924
          CIP

©1999 John Haugse
ISBN 1-55874-677-3

Publisher: Health Communications, Inc.
          3201 S.W. 15th Street
          Deerfield Beach, FL 33442-8190

Cover and inside illustrations by John Haugse
Cover redesign by Larissa Hise
Book design by Lawna Patterson Oldfield

Dedicated to the women and men working in nursing homes,
for their commitment to the service of others.

Contents

Acknowledgments

Special thanks to **Melissa Marsland**, whose editorial collaboration helped shape this project and whose faith and perseverance kept it on track.

To **Helen Byers**, for her enthusiastic support and editing.

To **Ruth Wolman**, for her many insights and careful eye.

To **Petra Mathers** and **Michael Mathers**, who first suggested that these drawings belonged in a book.

To my agent, **Anne Depue**, for her input and advice.

To **Terry Melton** and **Nancy Combs**, who read every script as though for the first time.

To my sister, **Ruth McKinney**, and my brother, **Bill Haugse**, for their love and support.

Introduction

One winter morning, I was walking with my father outside his nursing home. It was snowing heavily. I glanced back to look at our trail and noticed that his tracks had almost vanished, while mine were still well defined. I joked with him about this and asked what he thought it meant. He replied, "I'm not surprised. I often feel like I'm disappearing."

Over the next six years, I watched as he lost one after another of the fragile connections that hold us to this world.

This is our story.

1

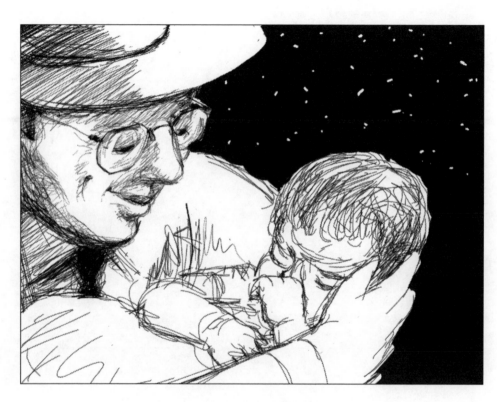

Starting Out

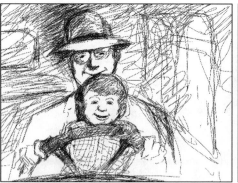

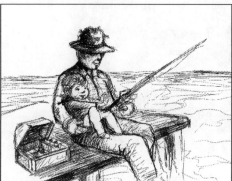

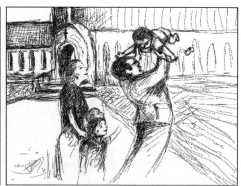

My father was a Lutheran minister.

He performed baptisms, weddings, funerals and wrote a new sermon every Friday.

He raised three children, coached a church basketball team . . .

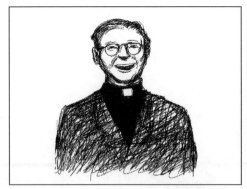

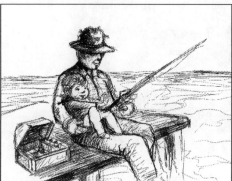

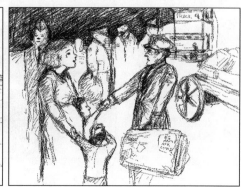

. . . and achieved the rank of Lt. Colonel in the Army Reserves.

There wasn't anything he couldn't do.

In 1943, he went off to war in the Pacific. I was five.

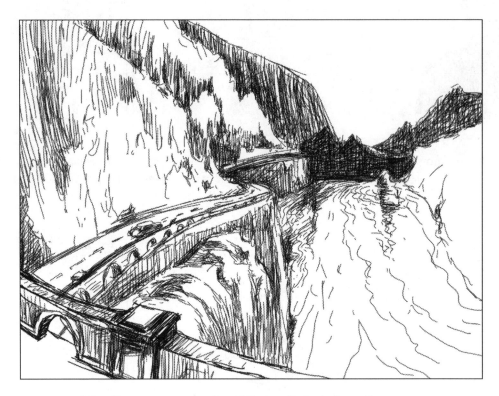

After the war, we moved out West and started our lives over.

As the years passed, the closeness I'd had with my father changed.

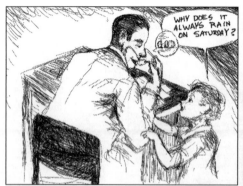 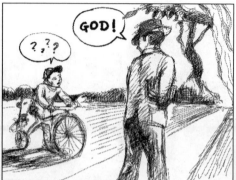 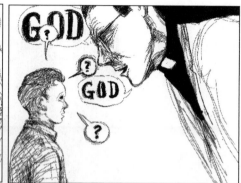

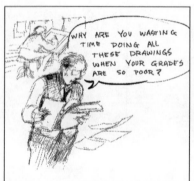 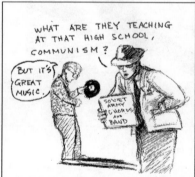 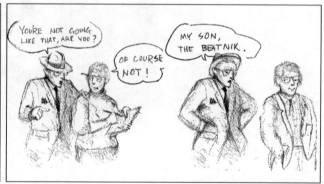

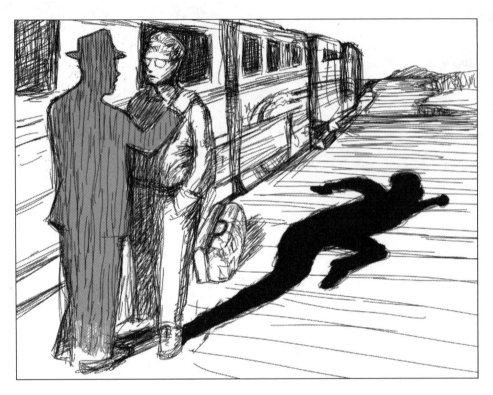

I left for college in 1956.

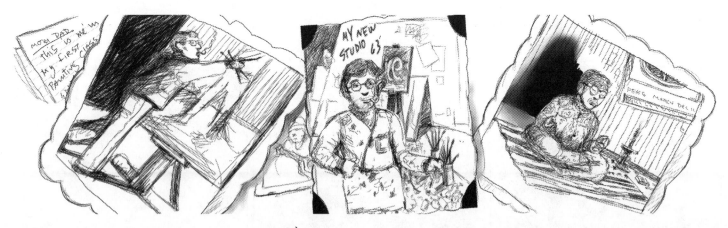

As soon as I could, I declared myself an art major.

After seven years of college and two degrees, I was painting full time and earning a meager living as a frame maker.

I learned Zen meditation, which my father referred to as part of an anti-Christ movement.

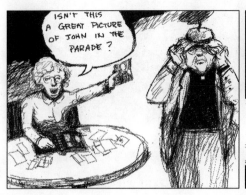

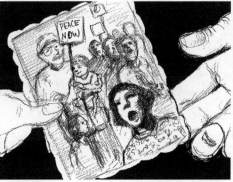

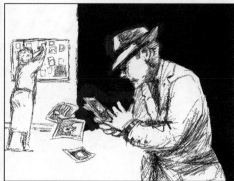

Starting Out

The distance between my father and me continued to grow until it seemed like
we were on opposite sides of every issue facing the country.

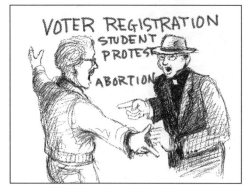 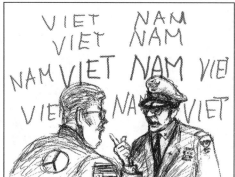 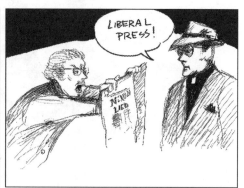

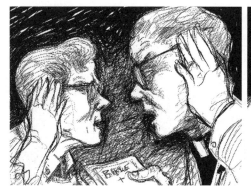 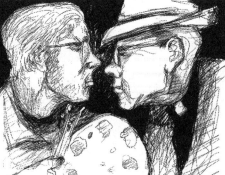 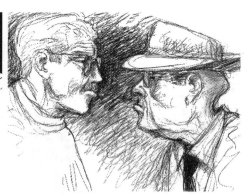

Over the years   we set our jaws and   lost sight of each other.

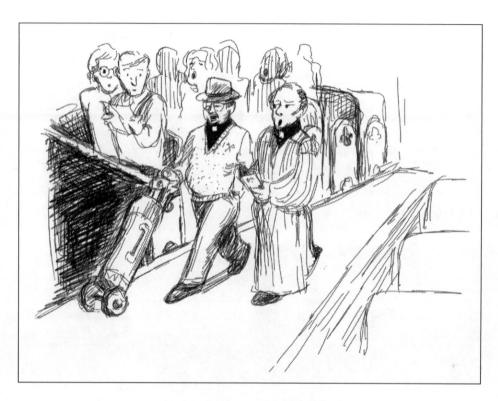

2

Signs of Trouble

Signs of Trouble

My father was in his late seventies when I first noticed that his memory was failing.
I accepted it as an annoying but normal part of his aging.

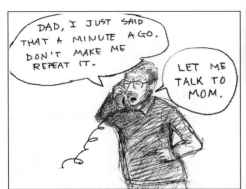

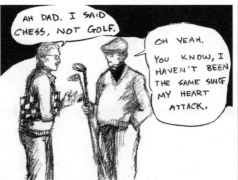

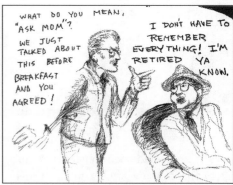

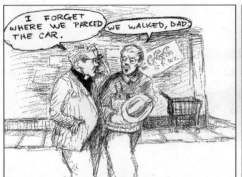

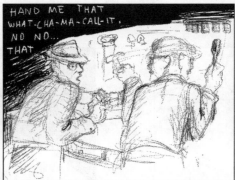

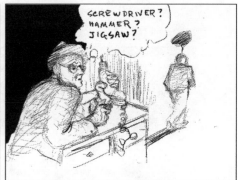

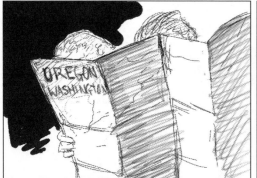

My wife and I had been considering moving to the Northwest. My folks lived in Washington, so we stayed with them while we looked for a place.

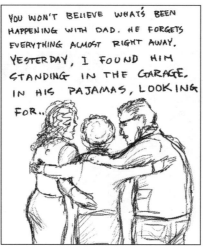

Mom was worried about Dad and wanted to talk.

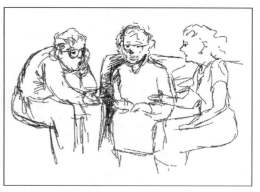

Whatever help we suggested was met with a gracious but firm refusal.

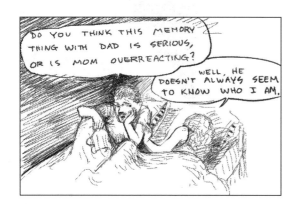

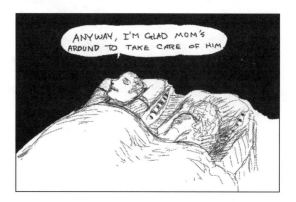

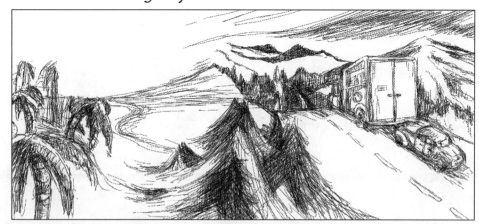

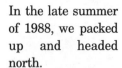 In the late summer of 1988, we packed up and headed north.

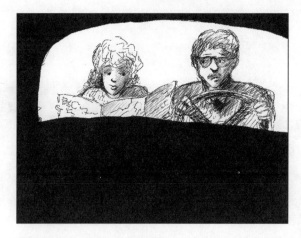

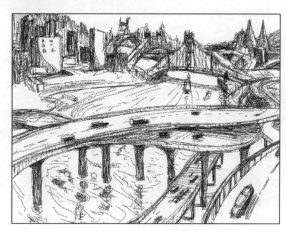

Although we didn't talk about it much, we knew that my parents were getting to the age when they would need more help and attention from us.

We moved to Portland, a two-hour drive from my parents' home in Washington.

Shortly after we settled in, I drove up to visit them. Mom sent Dad and me on an errand.

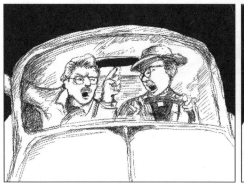

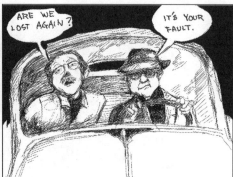

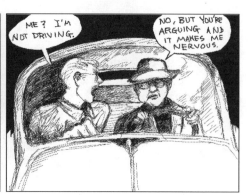

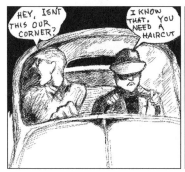

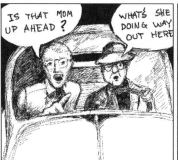

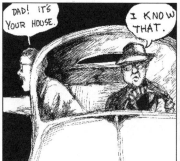

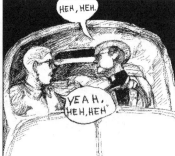

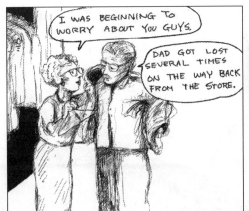

I WAS BEGINNING TO WORRY ABOUT YOU GUYS.

DAD GOT LOST SEVERAL TIMES ON THE WAY BACK FROM THE STORE.

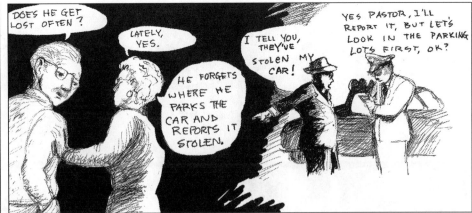

DOES HE GET LOST OFTEN?

LATELY, YES.

HE FORGETS WHERE HE PARKS THE CAR AND REPORTS IT STOLEN.

I TELL YOU, THEY'VE STOLEN MY CAR!

YES PASTOR, I'LL REPORT IT, BUT LET'S LOOK IN THE PARKING LOTS FIRST, OK?

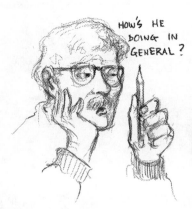

HOW'S HE DOING IN GENERAL?

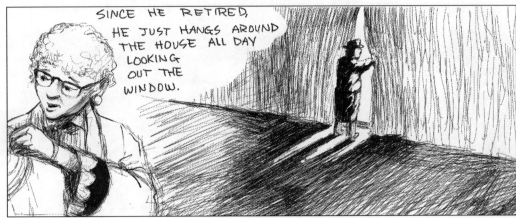

SINCE HE RETIRED, HE JUST HANGS AROUND THE HOUSE ALL DAY LOOKING OUT THE WINDOW.

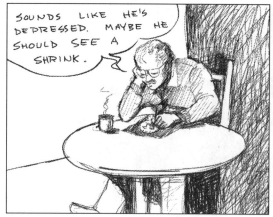

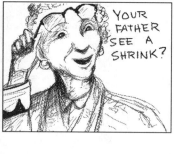

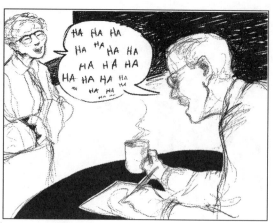

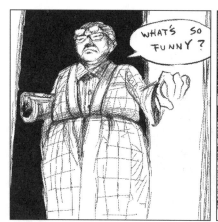

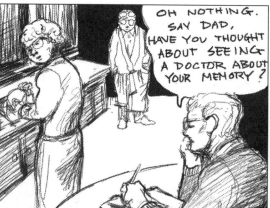

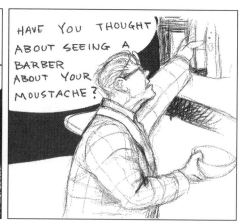

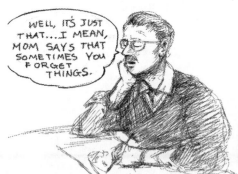

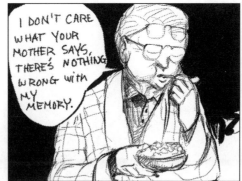

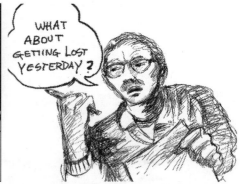

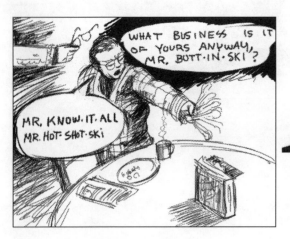

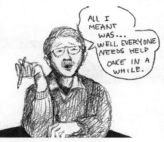

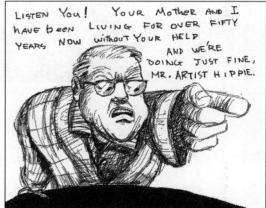

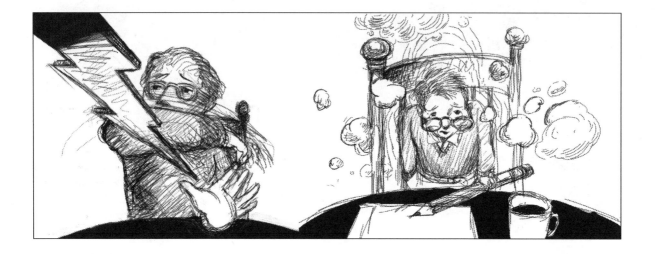

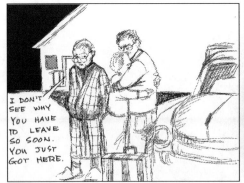

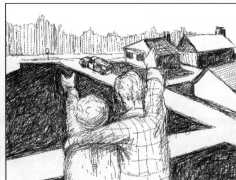

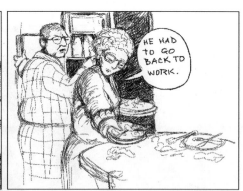

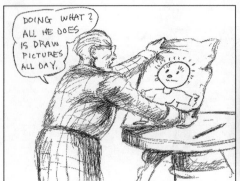

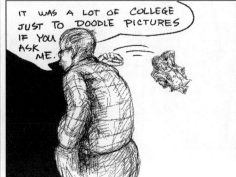

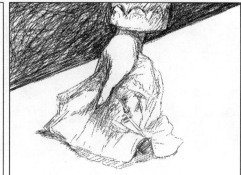

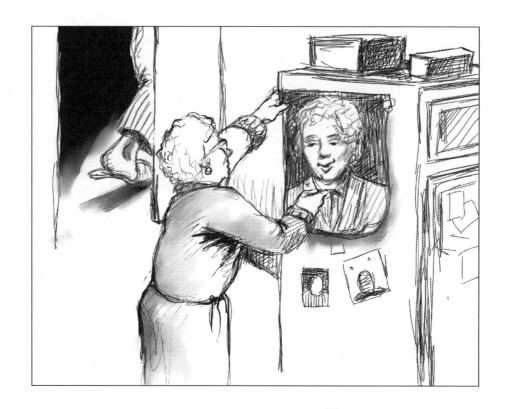

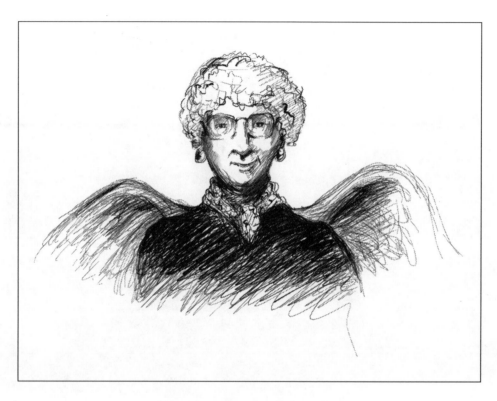

3

Mom Steals Home

I was working late on an animation assignment when I got a call from Dad.

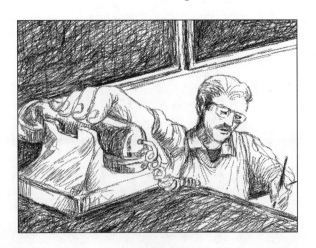
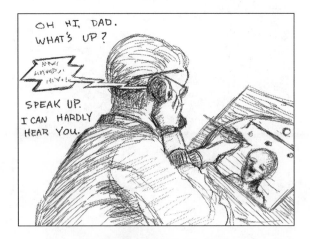
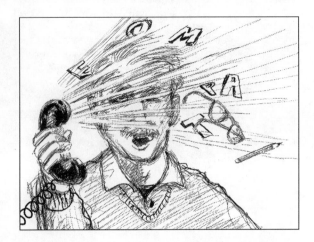
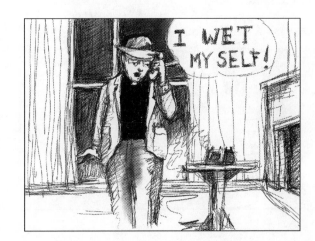

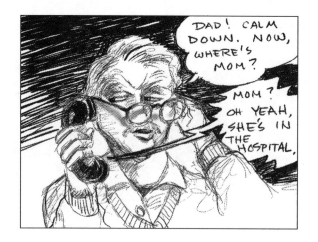

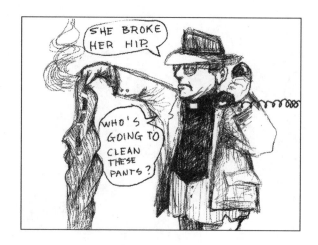

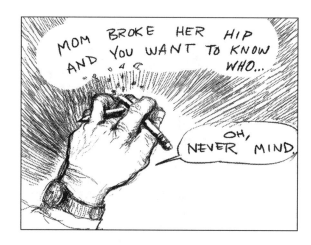

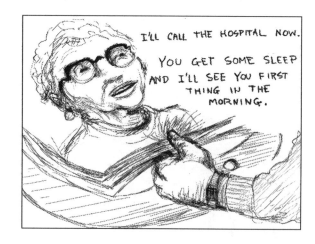

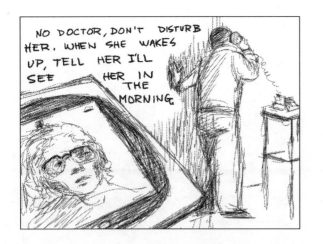

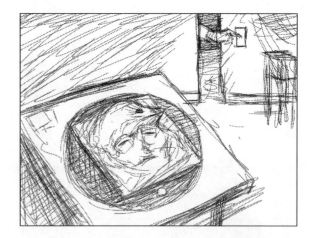

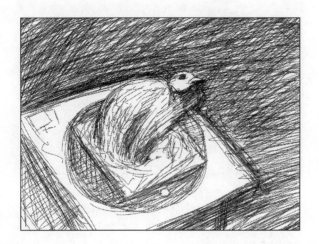

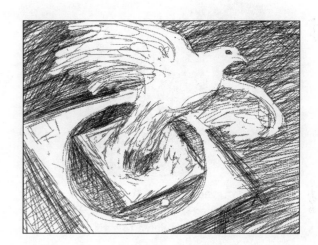

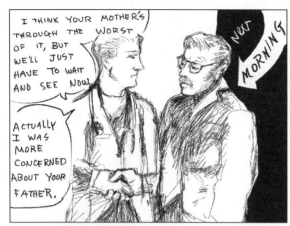

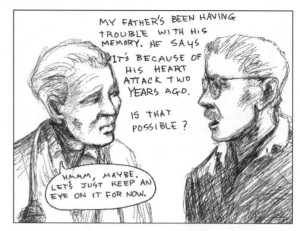

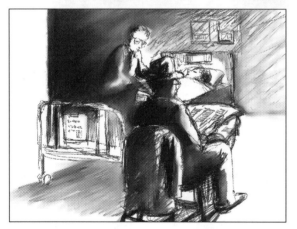

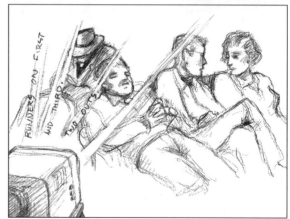

Late that afternoon, Mom took a turn for the worse. I called my brother Bill and sister Ruth and settled down to wait.

By the time everyone got to the hospital, Mom's condition was critical. We took turns grabbing naps. A baseball game blared on the television in the waiting room.

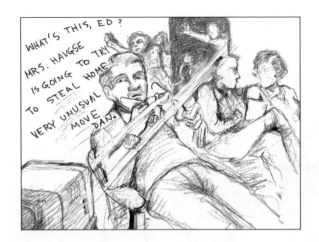

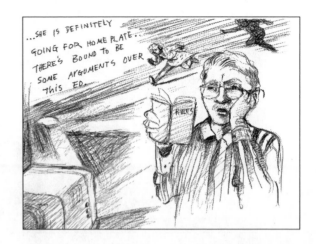

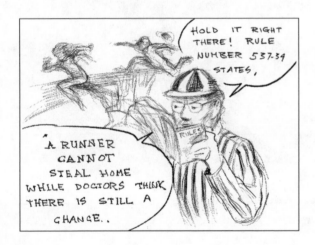

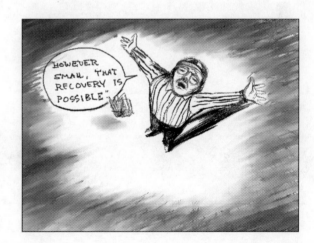

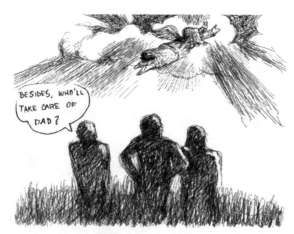

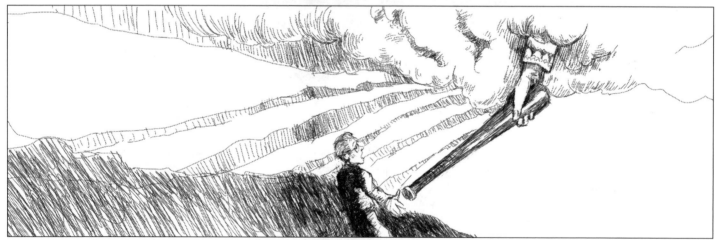

BATTER
UP

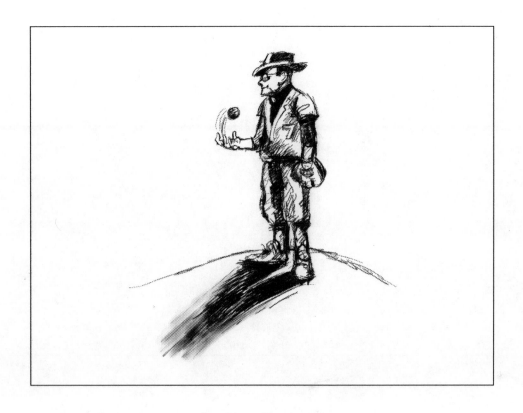

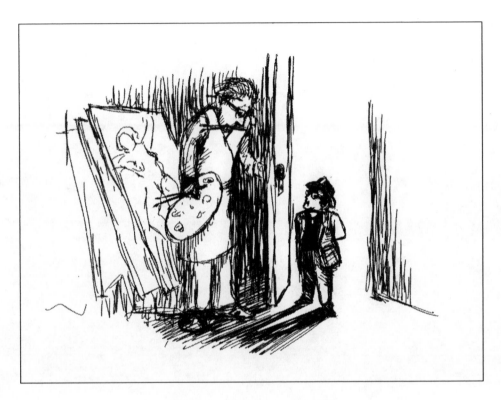

4

Who Gets Dad?

The Funeral

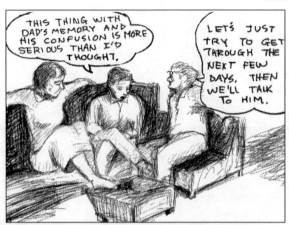

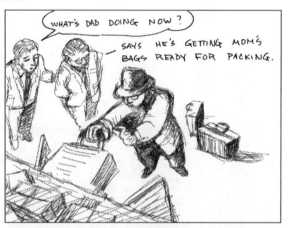

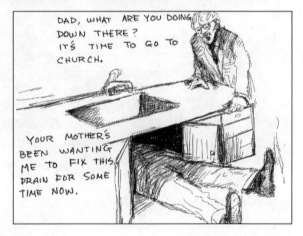

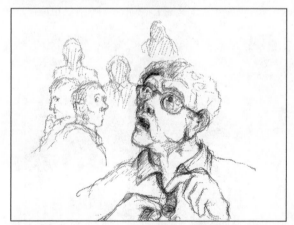

Moments before we were to leave for the funeral,
Dad thought he was suffering a heart attack.

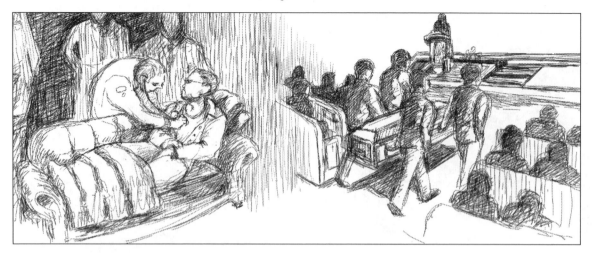

The funeral was held without Dad.

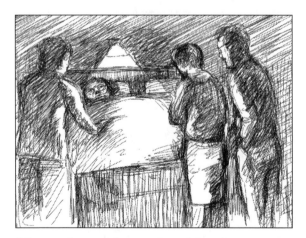

His attack turned out to be a false alarm.

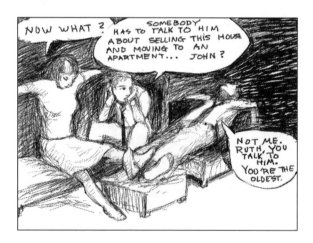

The next morning.

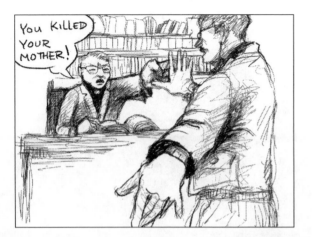

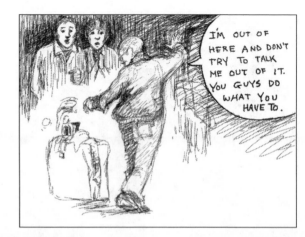

Ruth and Bill stayed on to help.

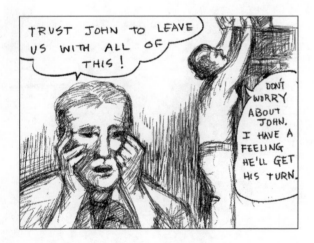

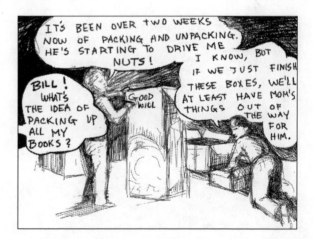

Dad's moods changed rapidly and without warning.

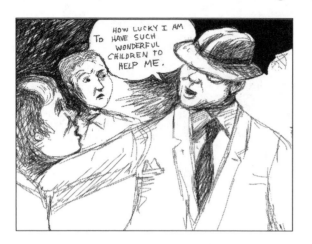

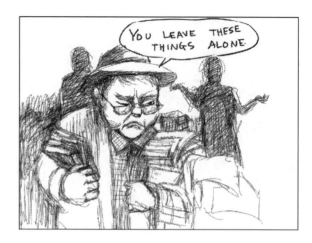

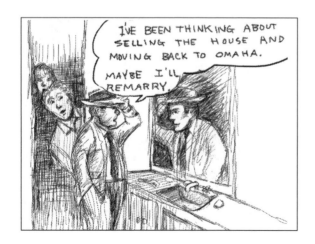

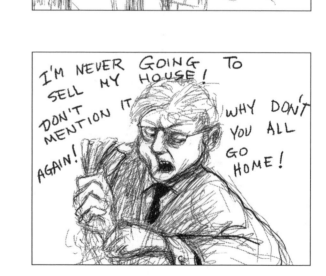

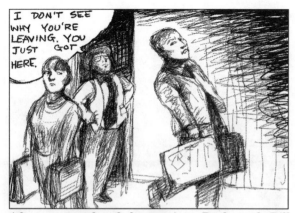

After a month of frustration, Ruth and Bill returned to their own lives.

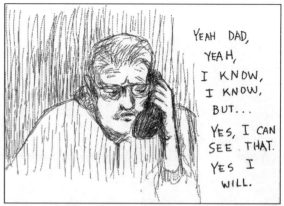

That evening Dad called to say he felt abandoned.

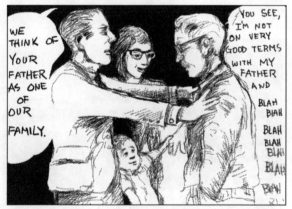

Worried that there was no one to look after him, I spoke to members of his church who assured me that they would take good care of him.

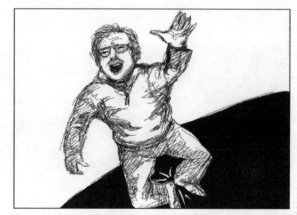

It was the perfect solution. I had absolved myself of responsibility by passing it on to others.

But I was wrong. Nothing is that easy.

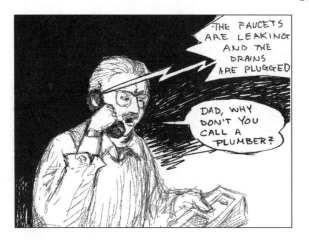

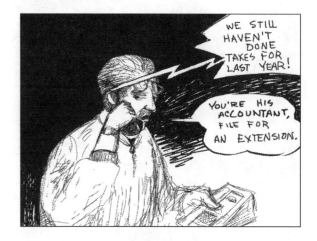

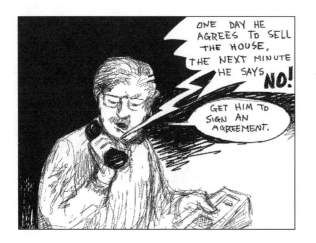

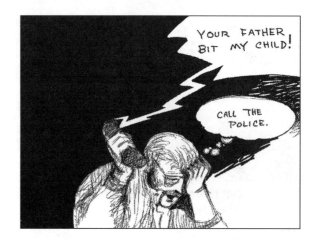

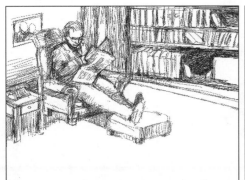 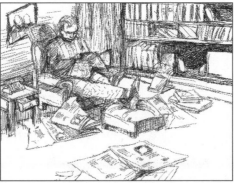 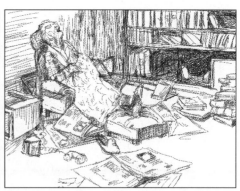

It became clear that Dad could not continue living in the house by himself.

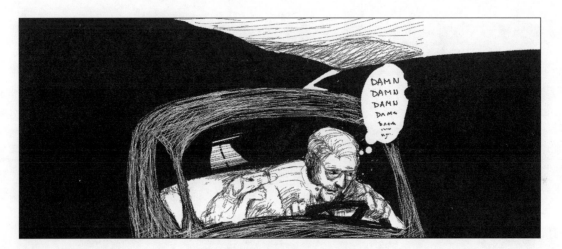

Eventually, I was drawn back in.

5

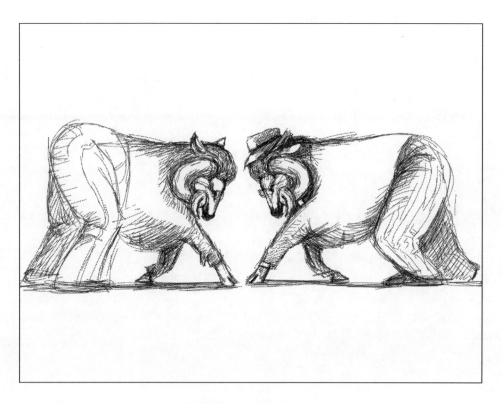

Taking Charge

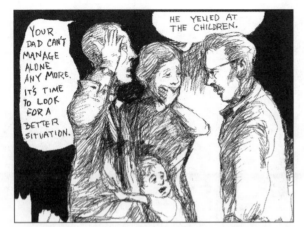

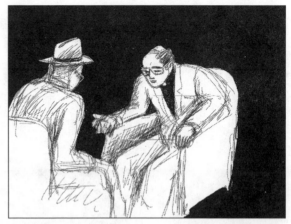

Nearly everyone spoke to him about selling the house, but it wasn't until the Bishop visited that he started to soften.

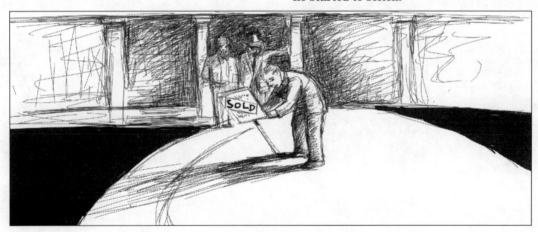

The house sold easily. Moving Dad was the hard part.

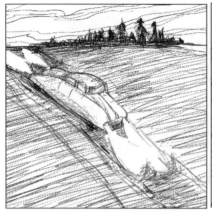
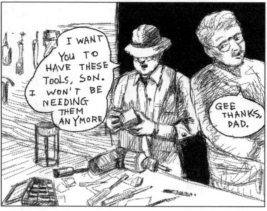
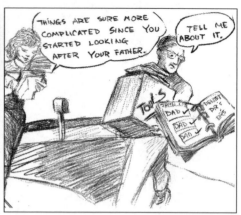

During those months I made many trips back and forth.

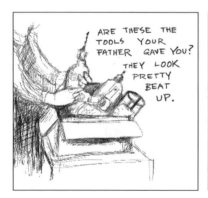
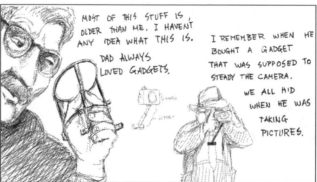
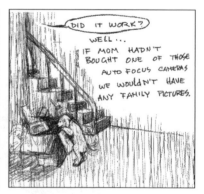

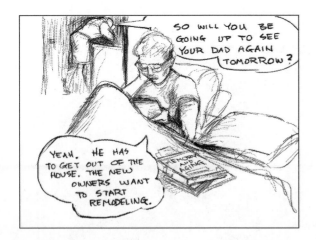

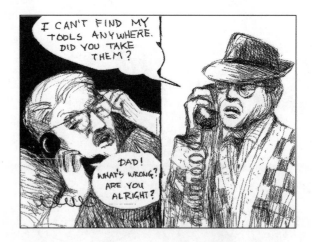

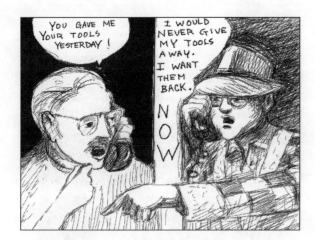

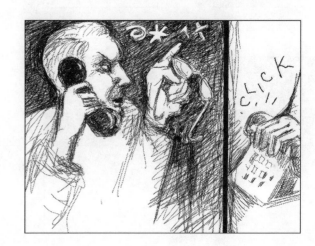

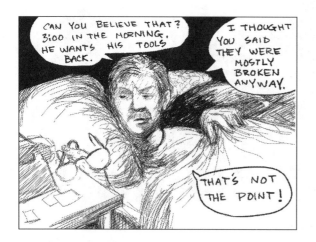

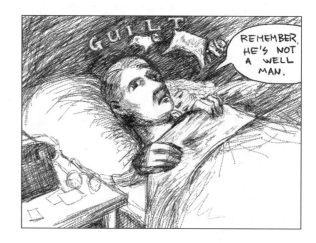

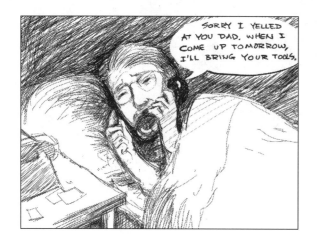

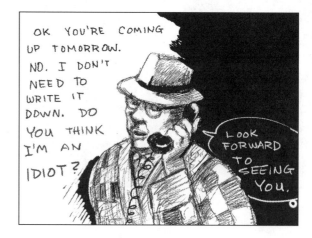

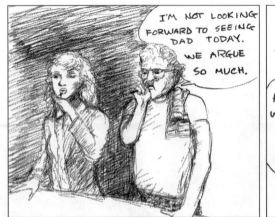

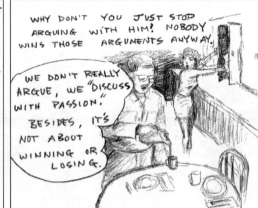

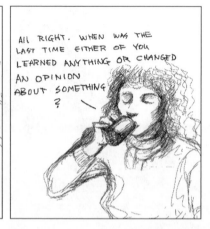

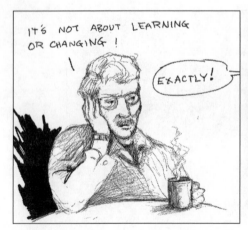

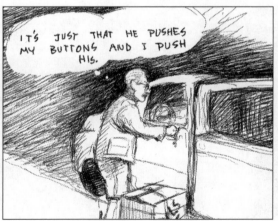

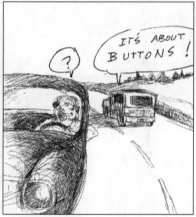

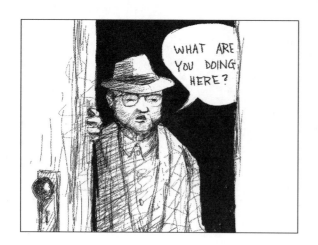

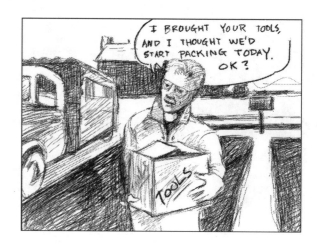

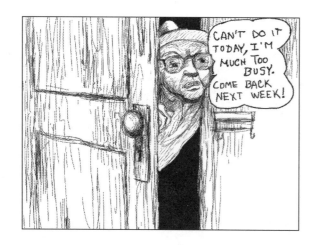

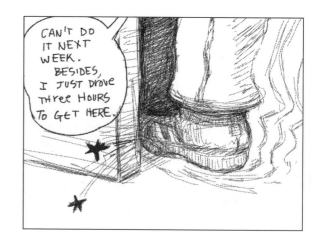

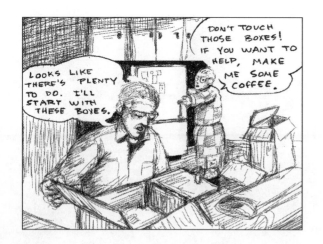

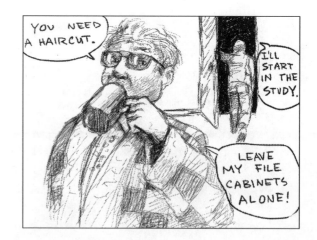

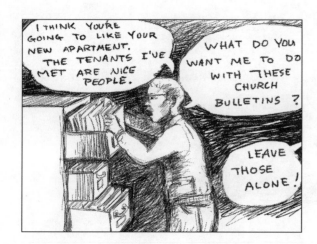

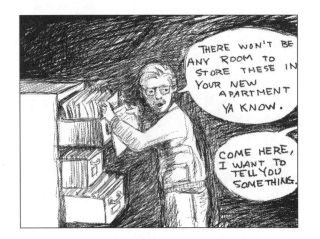

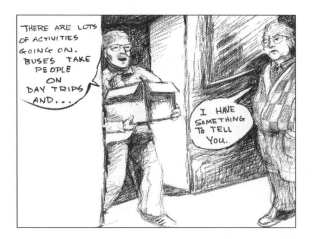

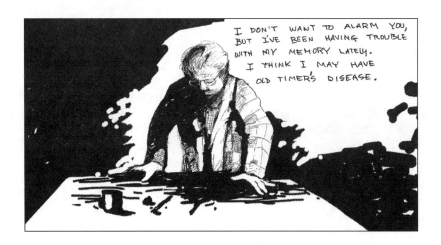

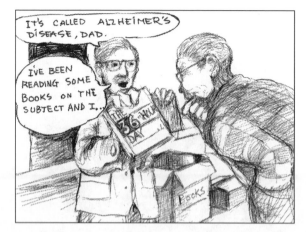

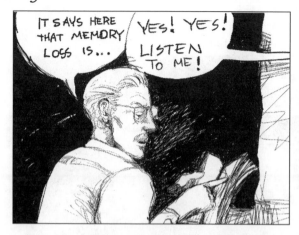

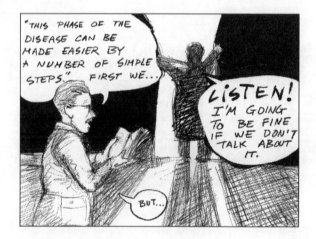

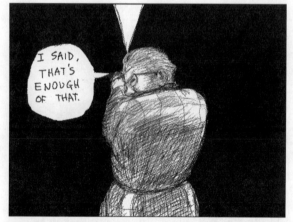

We never mentioned his memory loss again or said the word *Alzheimer's*.

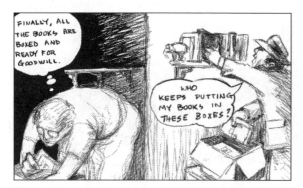

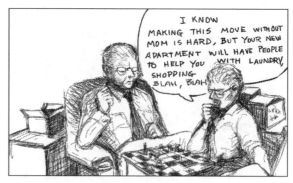

We had wanted to get Dad into an assisted living environment, but he wouldn't hear of it. Instead we found space for him in a retirement community with nursing aides on staff.

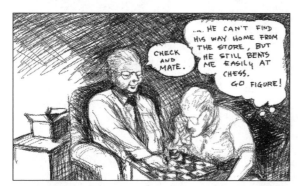

Realizing that Dad would never willingly move out of his house, I took a few of his things to the new apartment and made it as homey as possible.

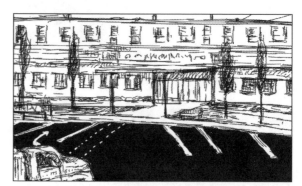

I drove him to his new home and introduced him to the staff. While they were settling him in, I went back to finish packing.

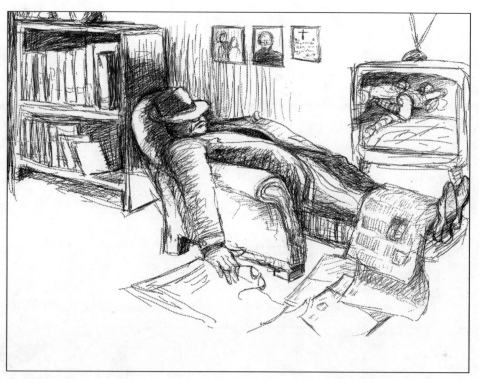

By the time I returned, Dad was asleep in his chair. He never mentioned the house again.

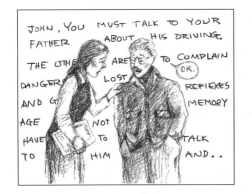

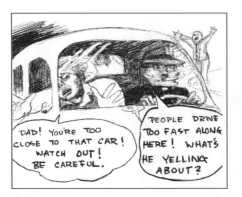

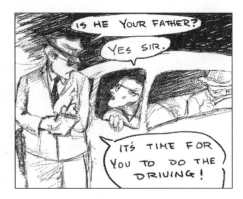

Dad's driving, which had been terrible for years, had become seriously dangerous. It seemed to me that everyone expected me to solve the problem.

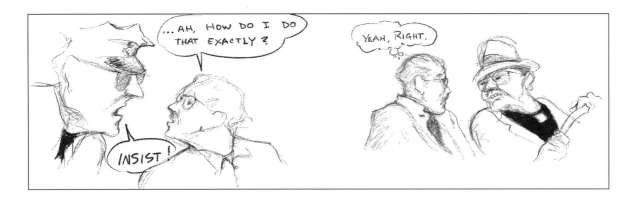

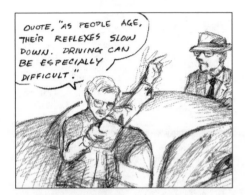

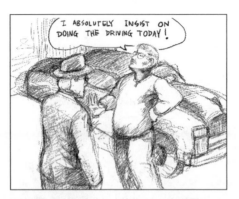

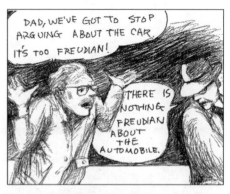

Reason: to think, form judgments and draw conclusions.

Confront: to face or oppose boldly.

Humor: to joke or amuse.

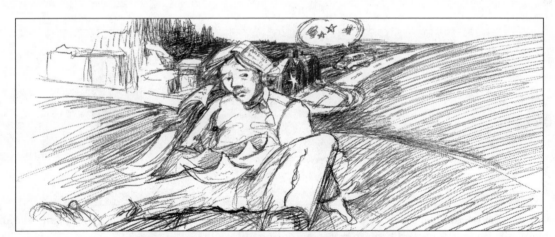

Frustrated: prevented from achieving an objective.

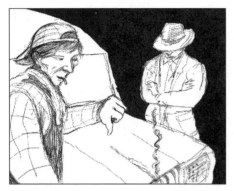

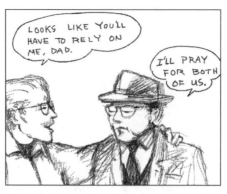

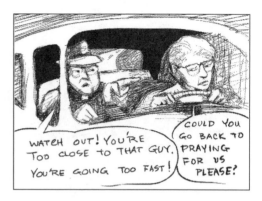

In the end, it was his mechanic who solved the problem by insisting he keep the car in the shop for "badly needed repairs."

Dad occasionally asked about the car, but he was easily distracted. I thought that perhaps he had wanted to stop driving, but hadn't known how.

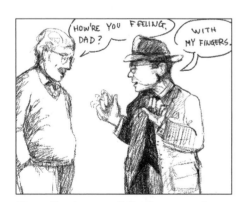

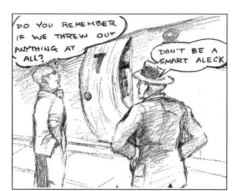

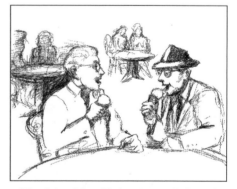

Once the issues of the house and car were resolved, Dad seemed to relax and be more like his old self. At times, I thought maybe the problem with his memory had been in my imagination, after all.

6

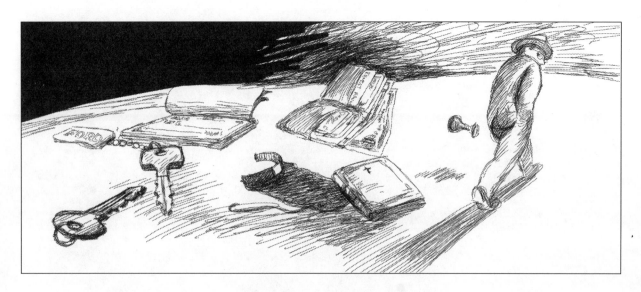

Losing Ground

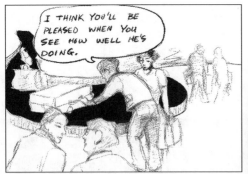

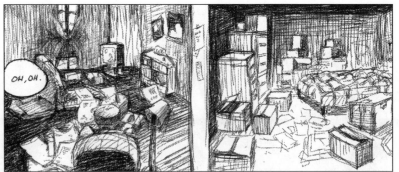

Several months later, my sister Ruth visited. I was eager for her to see how well Dad was doing in his new living arrangements.

Somehow, he had managed to get all his boxes out of storage and into his apartment.

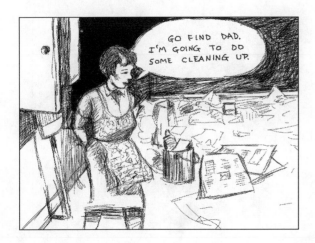

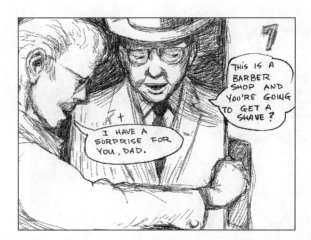

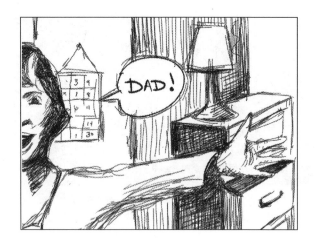

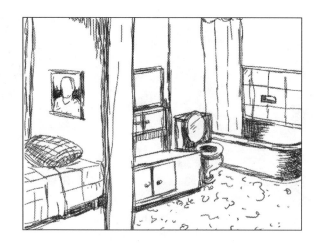

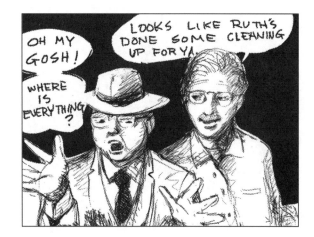

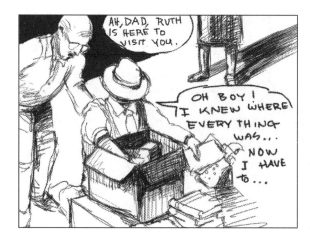

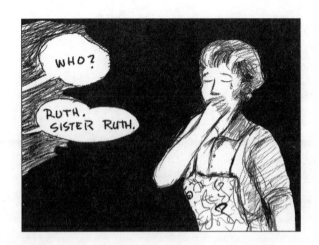

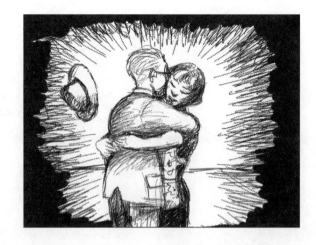

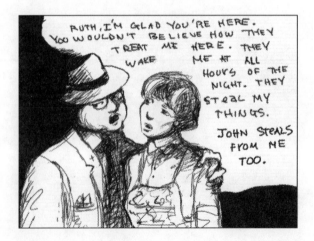

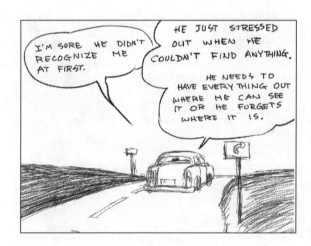

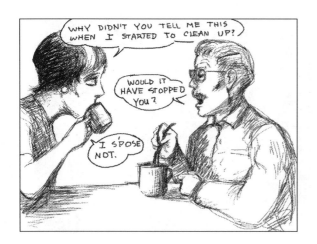

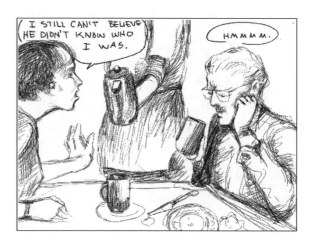

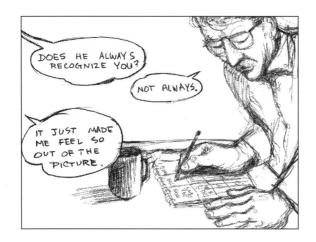

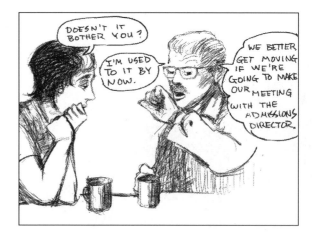

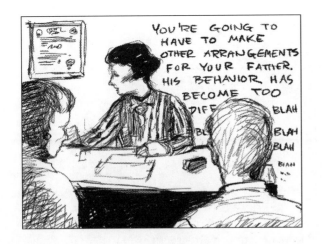

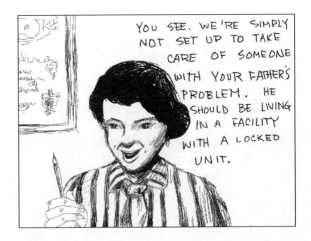

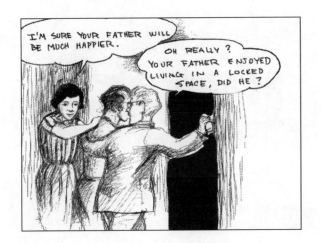

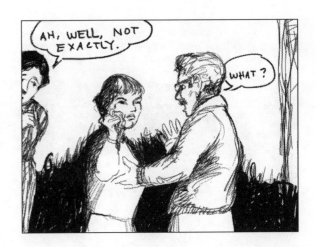

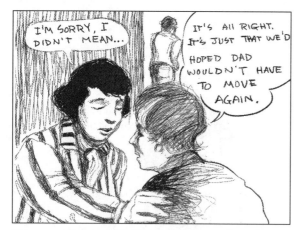

Once again, we had to find another living
arrangement for Dad. The first step was a doctor's evaluation.

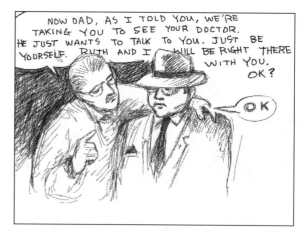

Dad agreed to see a doctor, but only on the condition that it be his cardiologist, a retired army
doctor now in private practice.

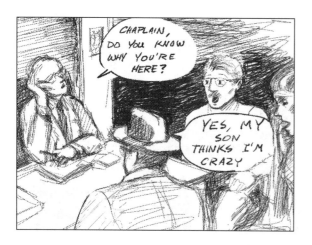

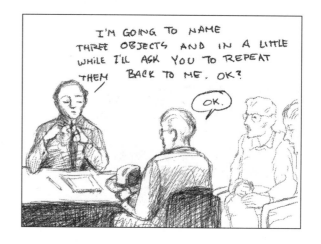

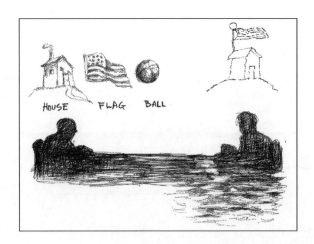

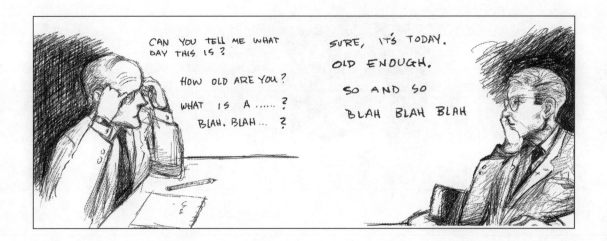

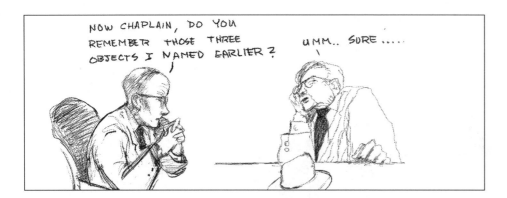

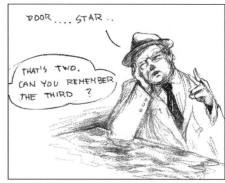

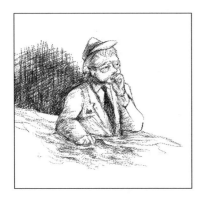

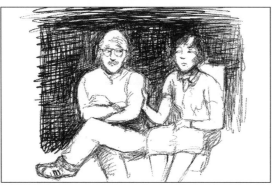

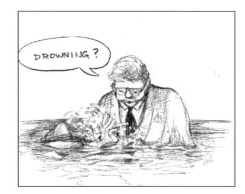

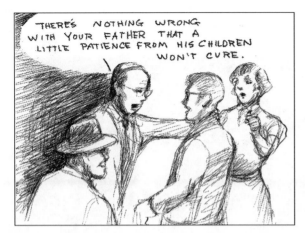

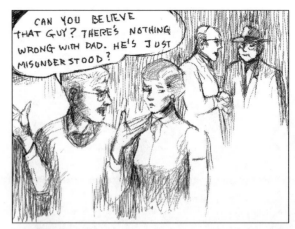

It's common for many doctors to view dementia as just part of aging. This happened a number of times before Dad was properly diagnosed.

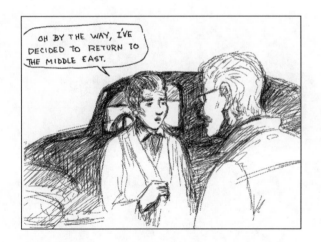

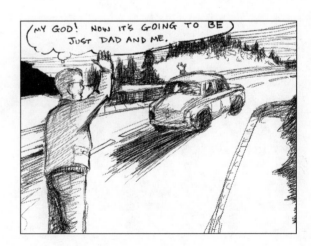

Since Ruth was planning to leave the country, I decided to look for a nursing home close to Portland.

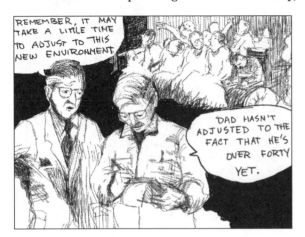

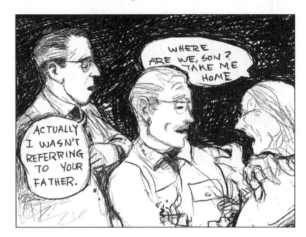

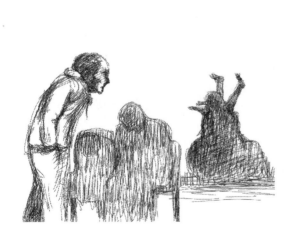

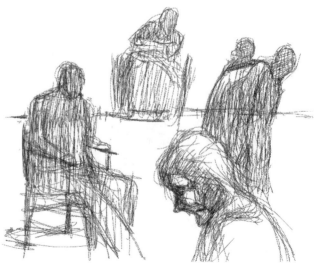

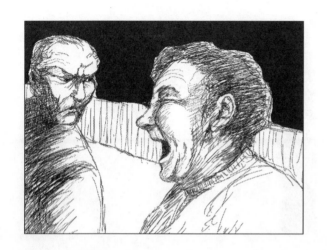

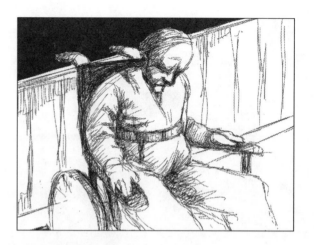

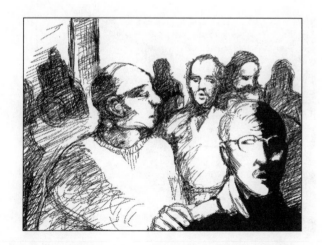

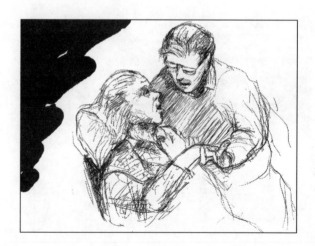

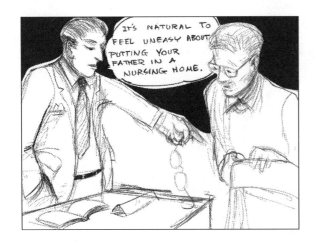

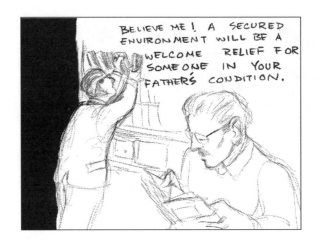

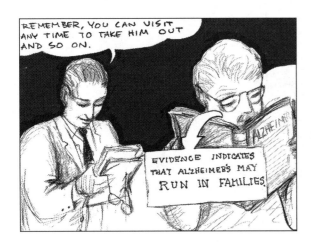

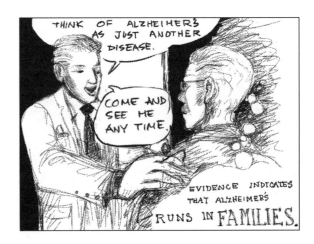

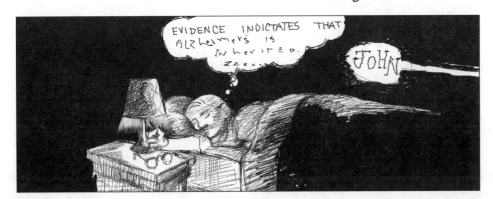

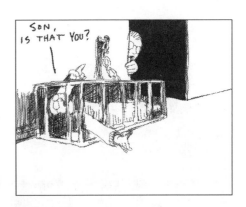

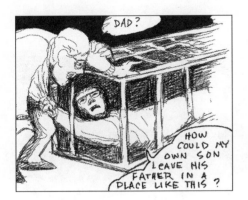

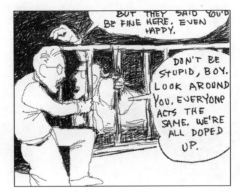

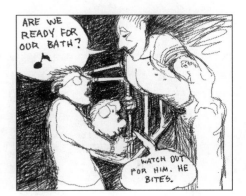

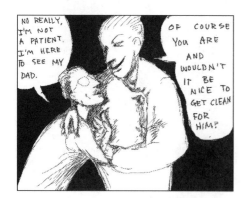

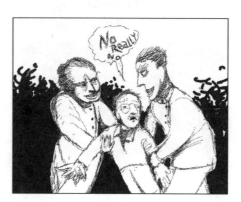

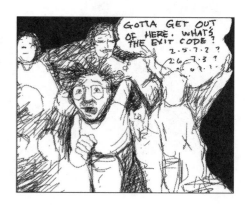

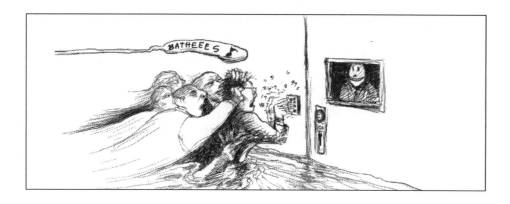

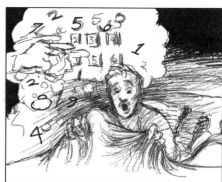

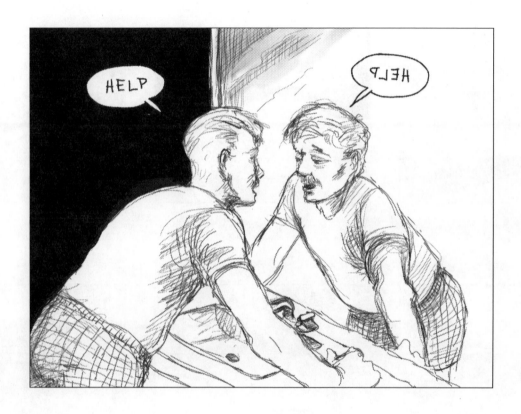

The next morning, I returned to the nursing home, determined to overcome my fear of this strange environment.

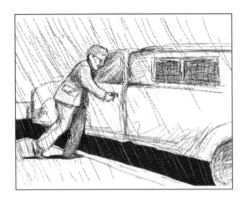

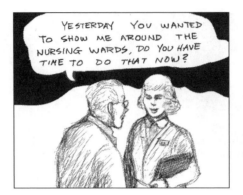

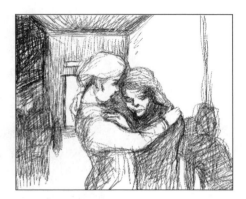

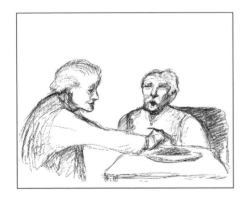

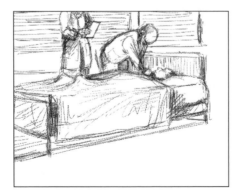

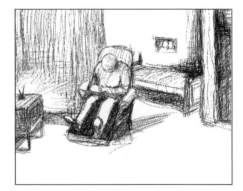

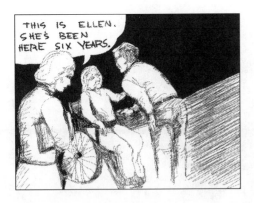

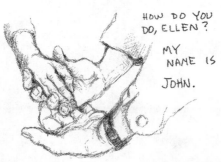

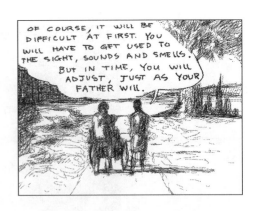

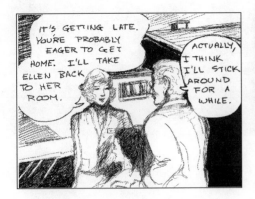

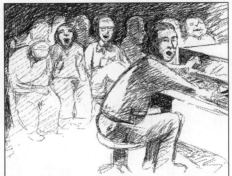

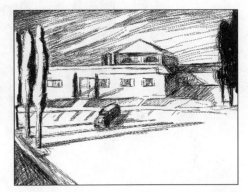

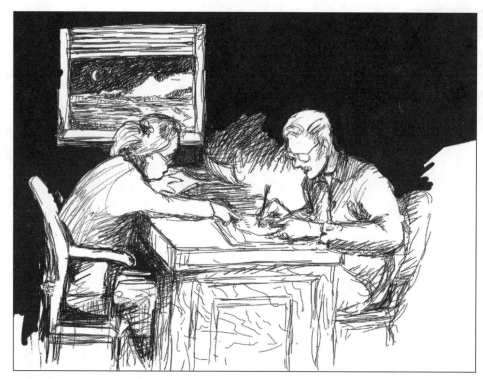

Late that evening, I signed the admittance papers.

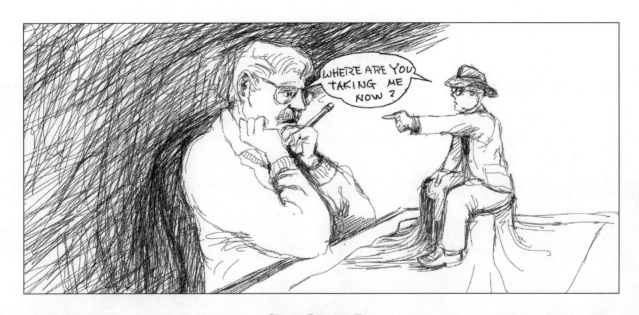

7

Settling In

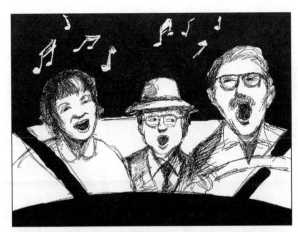

Ruth and I moved Dad to his new home outside Portland. We were all in good spirits and sang the whole way.

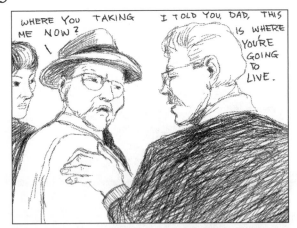

But, when we got to the nursing home, Dad's mood turned ugly.

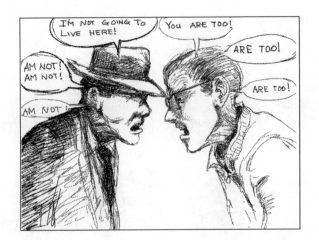

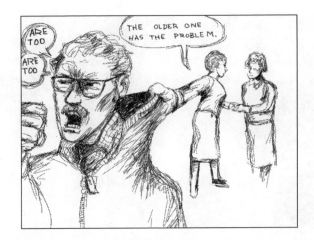

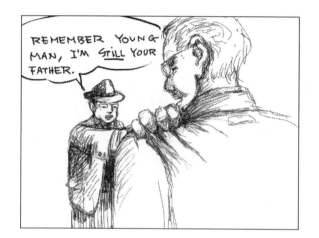

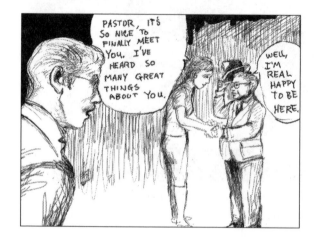

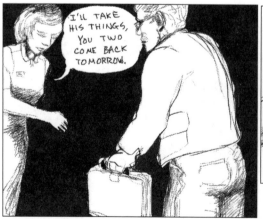

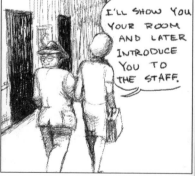

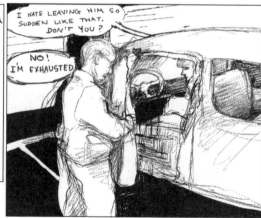

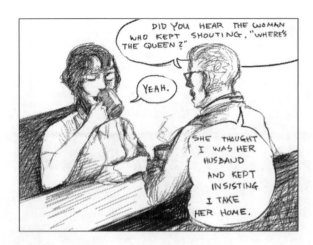

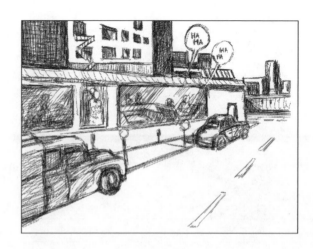

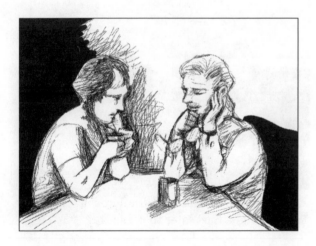

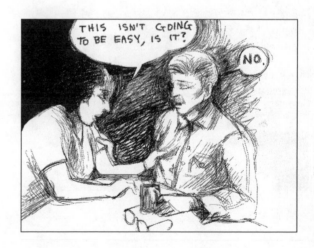

The next morning, we finished clearing out Dad's apartment.

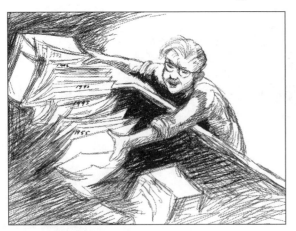

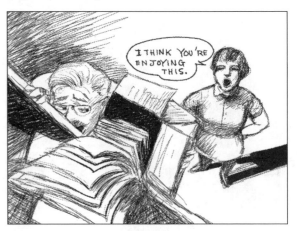

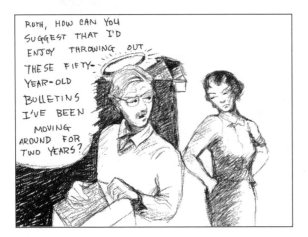

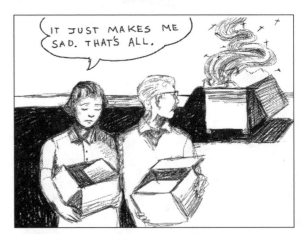

Ruth returned to Seattle that afternoon. She left for the Middle East later that month.

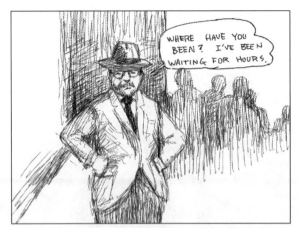
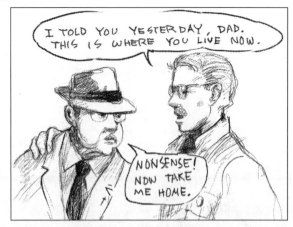

When I got to the nursing home the next morning, Dad was waiting for me at the door.

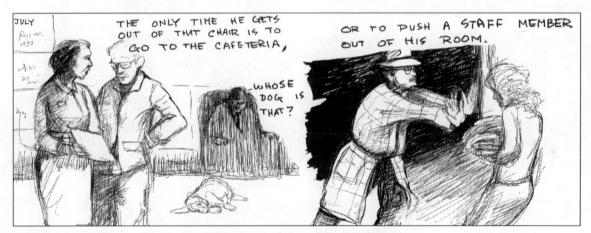

His anger continued for months.

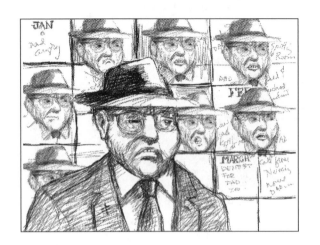

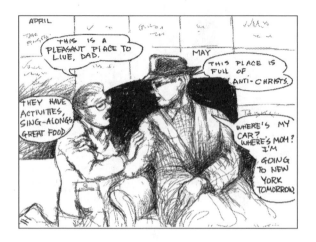

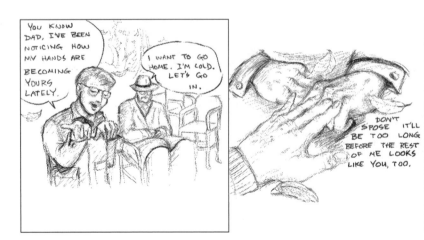

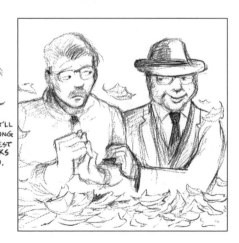

Dad slowly accepted his situation, and we settled into a routine.

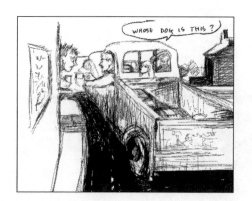

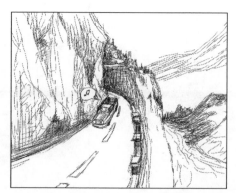

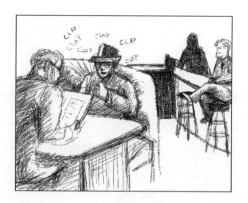

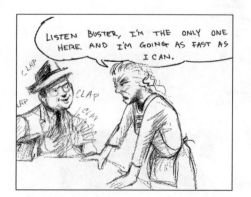

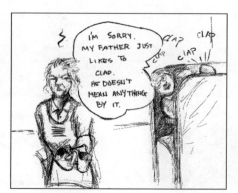

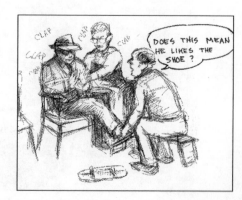

We began to build a new relationship based on my early childhood memories.

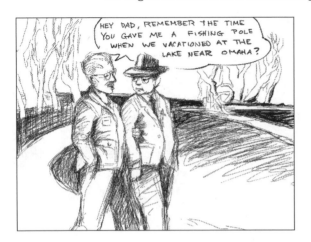

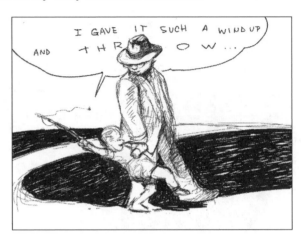

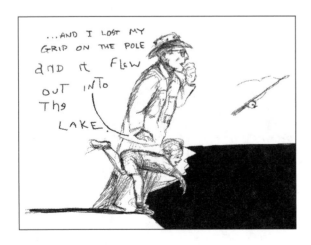

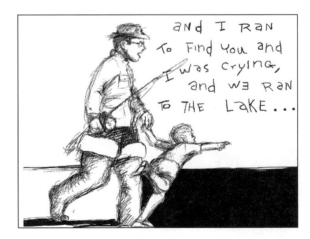

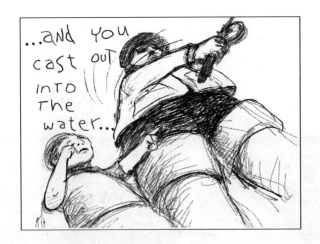

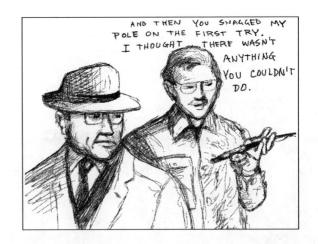

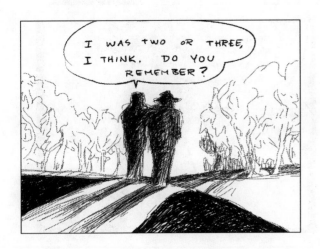

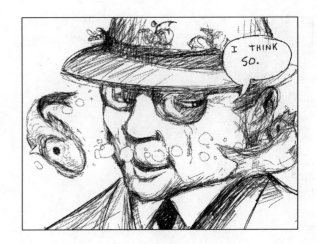

During this time, I talked to Dad in a way I had never been able to before. He just whistled or clapped his hands and watched me intently.

But there were always surprises.

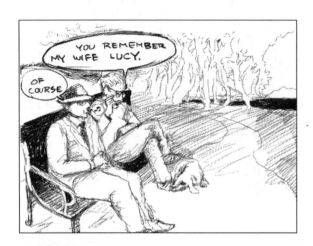

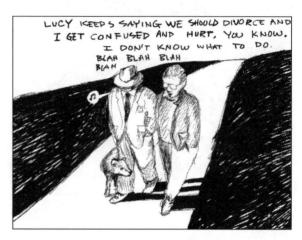

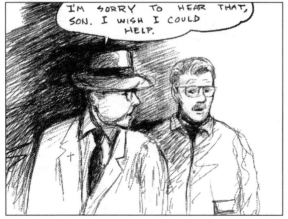

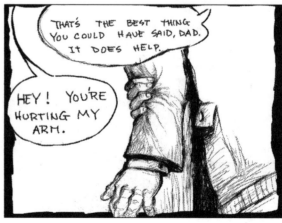

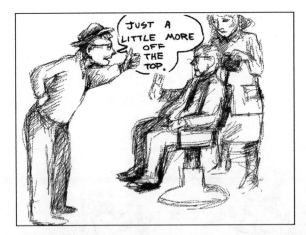

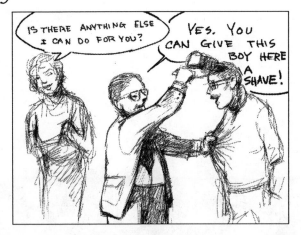

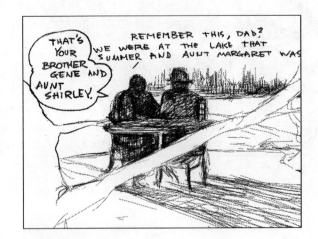

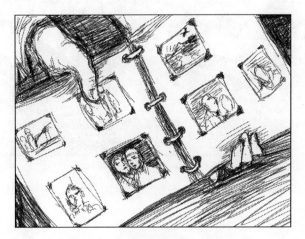

Remember?

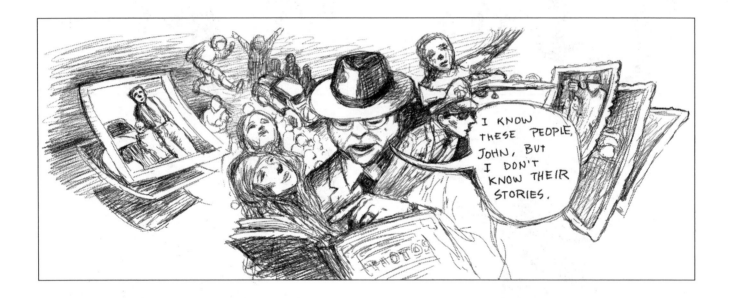

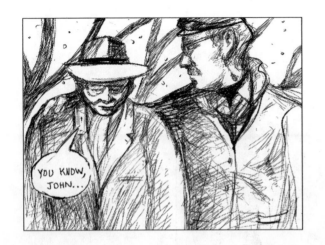
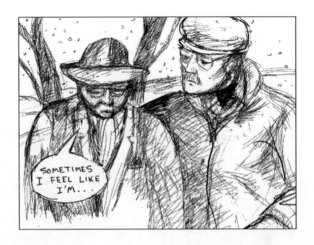
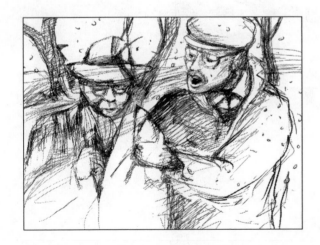
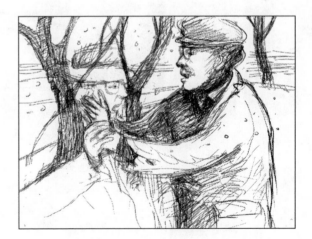

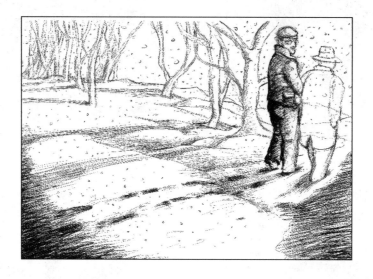

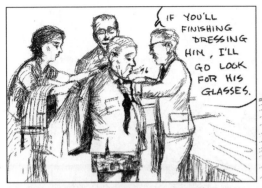

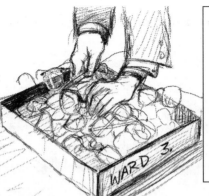

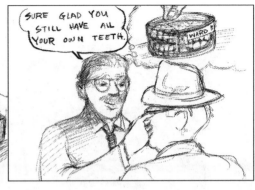

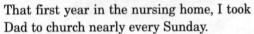

That first year in the nursing home, I took Dad to church nearly every Sunday.

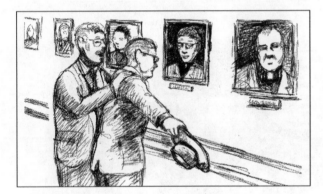

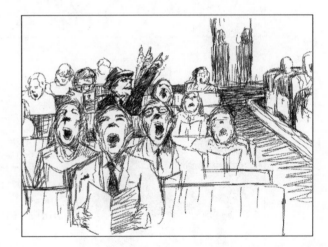

A highlight of going to church was stopping and looking at his picture in the entry. He had helped to organize this church and was its first ordained minister over forty years before.

Coffee hour after church was part of our routine.

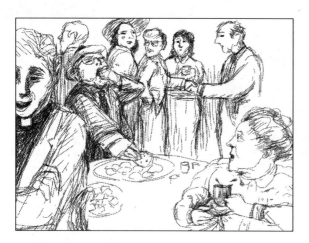

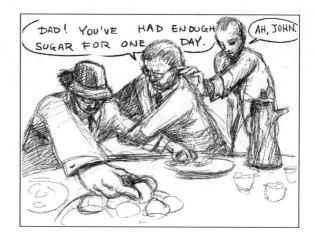

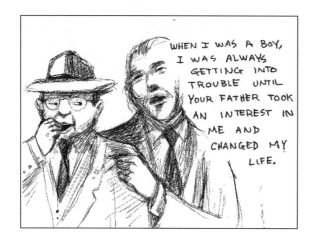

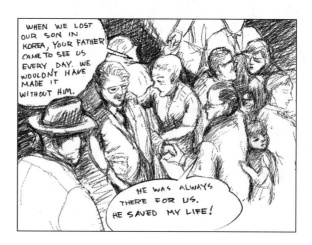

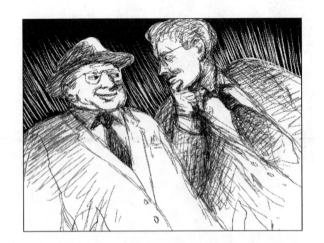

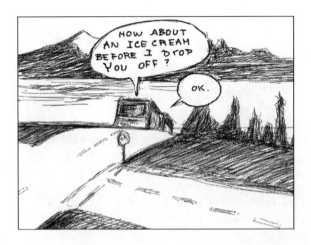

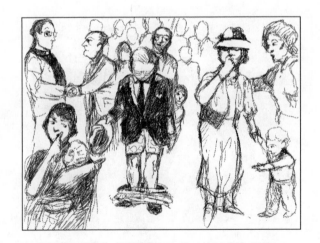

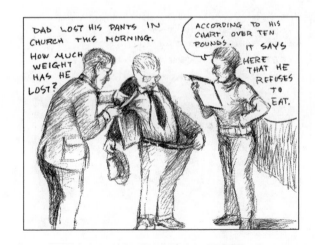

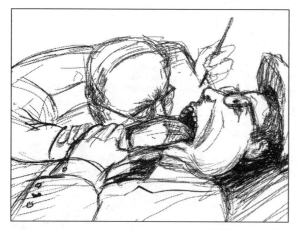

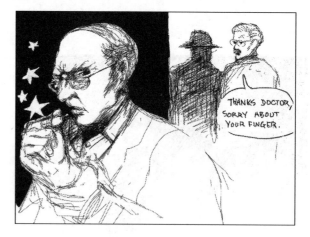

The next morning, a dentist pulled a badly impacted molar. Dad regained his weight in no time.

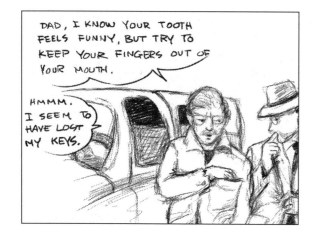

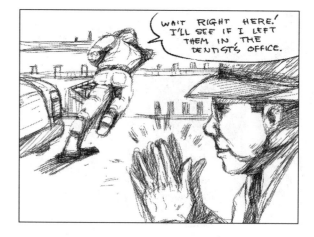

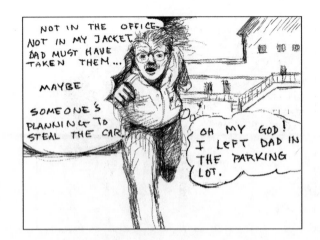

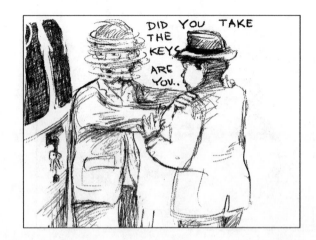

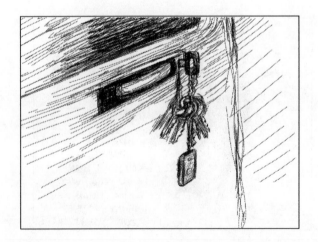

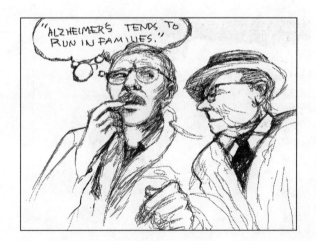

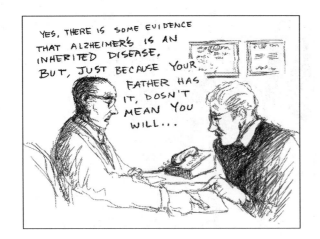

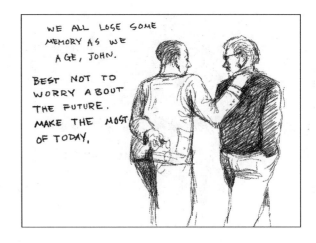

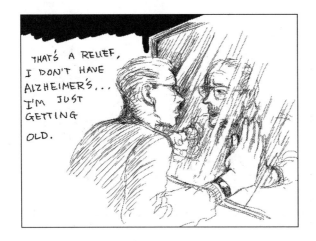

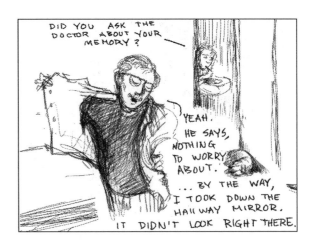

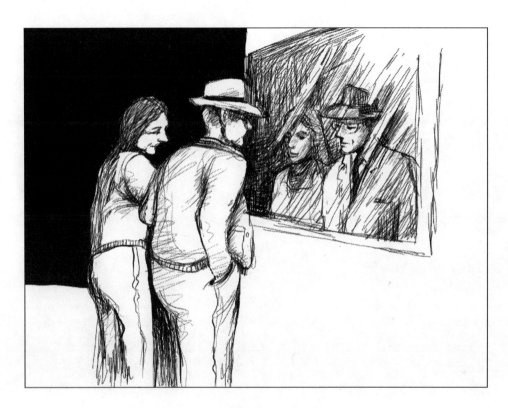

8

Susan

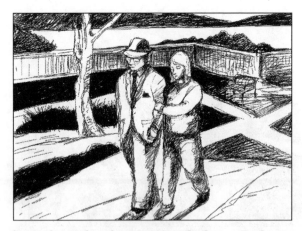

Several months after entering the home, Dad met Susan. She was in her early seventies and also suffered from Alzheimer's disease. They became convinced that they were married.

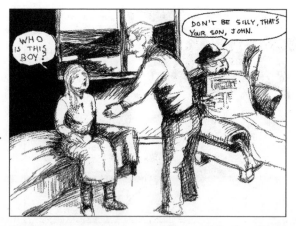

Susan never remembered me, so we had a ritual introduction on each visit.

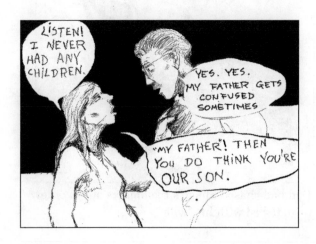

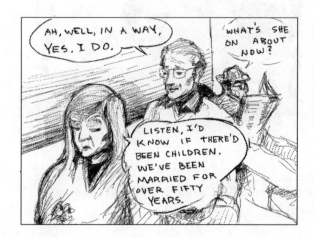

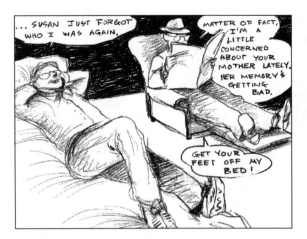

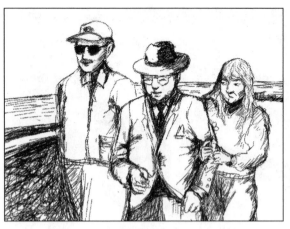

For a while Susan joined us on our walks, although she was always suspicious of me.

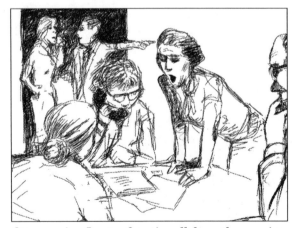

One evening I got a frantic call from the nursing staff.

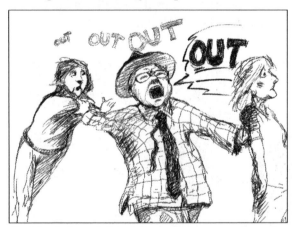

Dad had chased Susan's roommates out in order to go to bed with his "wife."

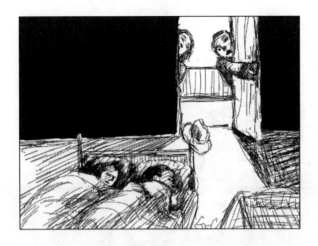

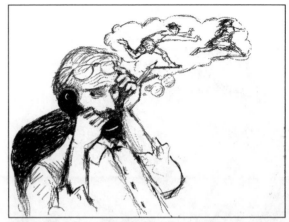

Naturally, I imagined the worst. We set up a meeting for the next morning.

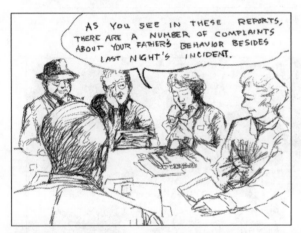

They showed me a long list of complaints about Dad's behavior.

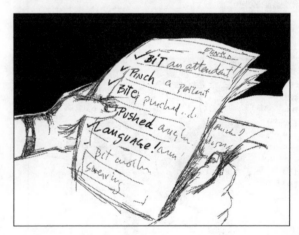

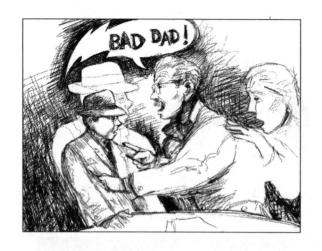

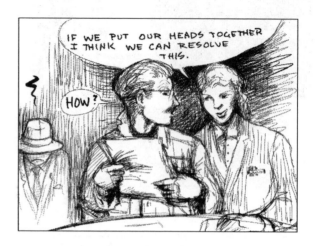

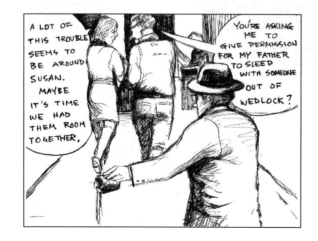

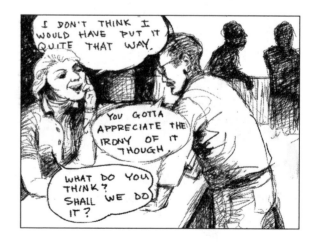

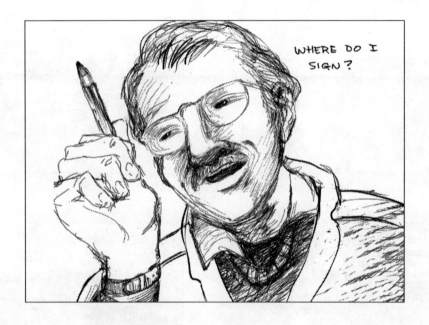

Before we had time to complete the paperwork, Dad got into more trouble.

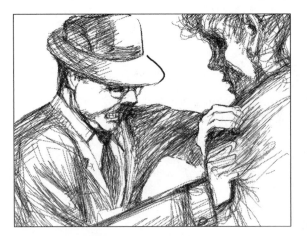

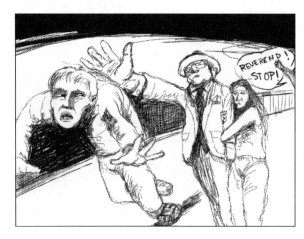

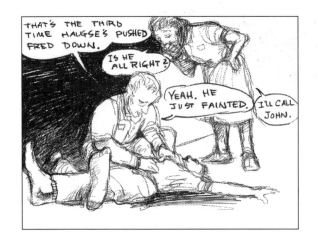

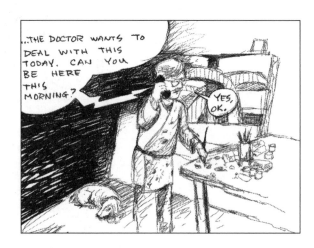

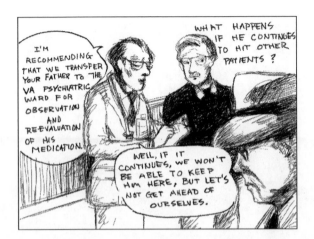

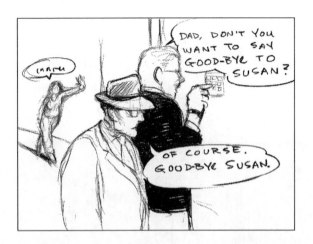

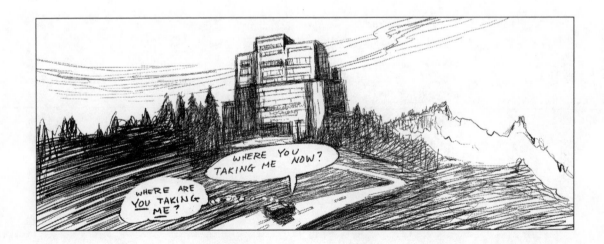

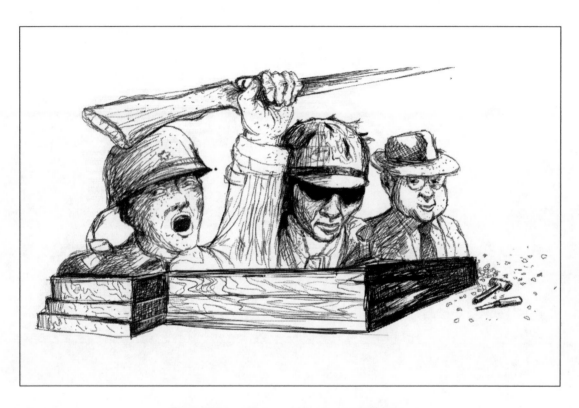

9

In the Company of Men

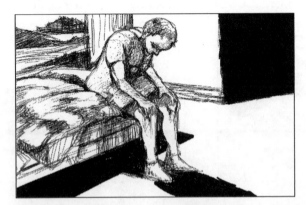 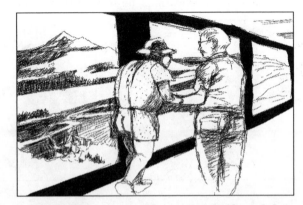

That first morning in the hospital, I was struck by how fragile Dad had become and how much he'd aged during the last few years. Those first days were difficult for both of us.

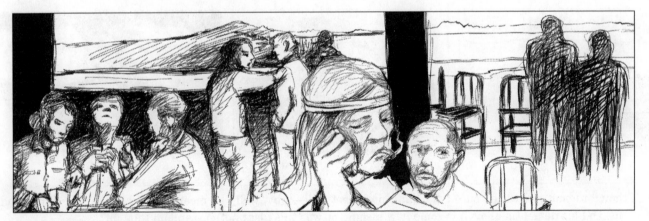

The VA psychiatric ward was very different from the nursing home, but Dad seemed to fit in easily.

Once off his medications, he seemed to get some of his humor back and started acting his old self again.

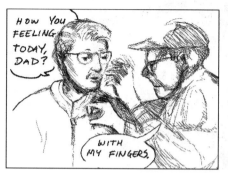 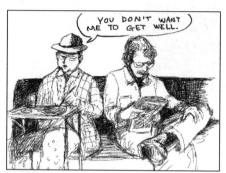 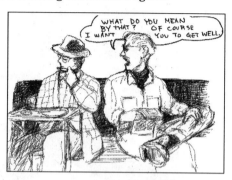

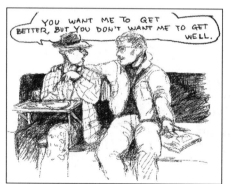 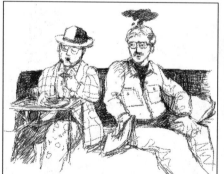 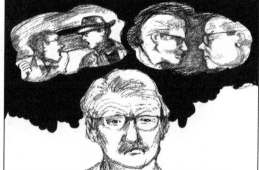

When I thought about it, I wasn't sure I did want him to get well—if by "well," he meant going back to how things had been between us. Did his dementia allow him some new insight, or was this just another random thought?

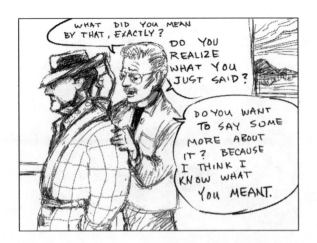

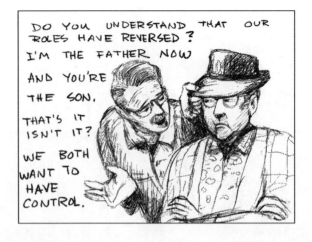

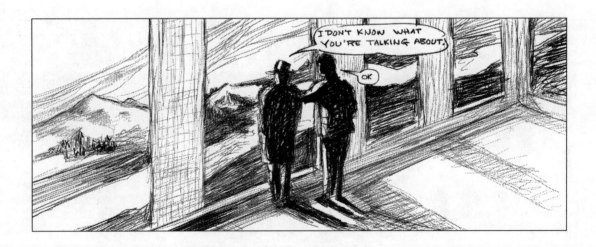

One evening while we were walking on the grounds of the VA hospital . . .

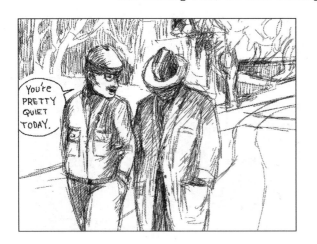

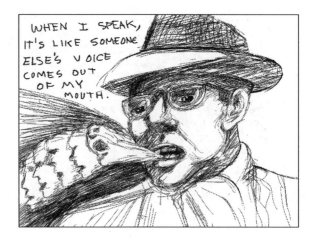

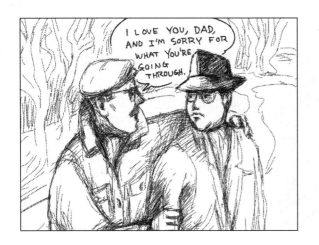

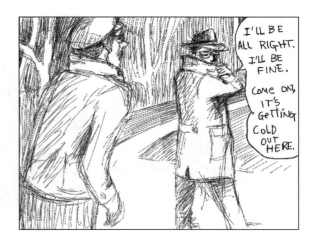

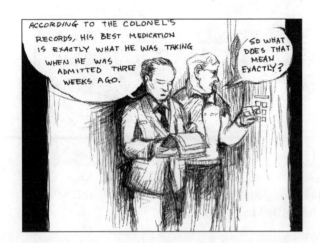

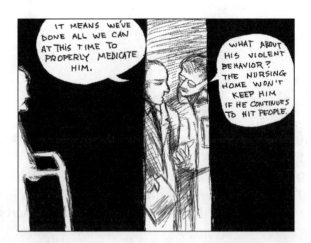

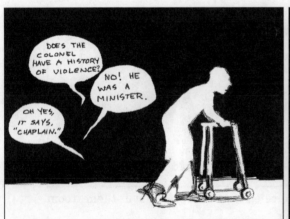

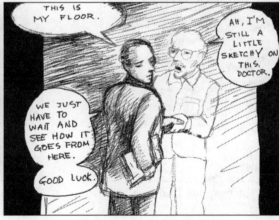

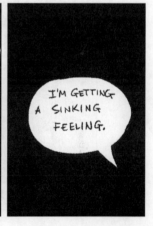

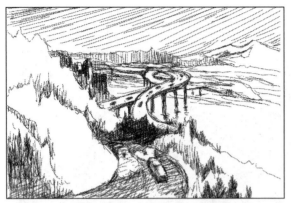 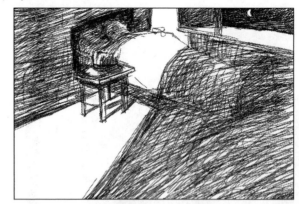

Dad was released later that evening. His medication was exactly what it had been when he came. I knew that if his violent behavior continued, I would have to find other living arrangements for him. The staff at the nursing home made him feel welcome, and in a short time he settled back in.

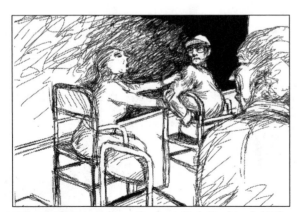 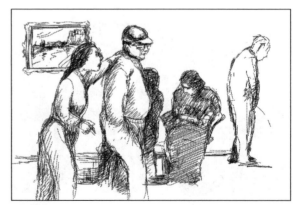

After his return from the hospital, Dad took little notice of Susan.

We canceled our plan to have them room together.

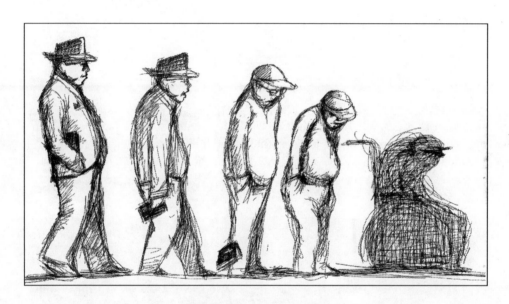

10

Sliding Home

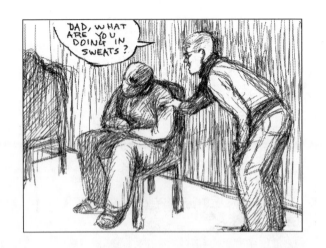

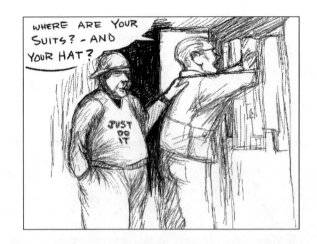

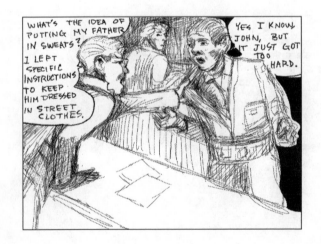

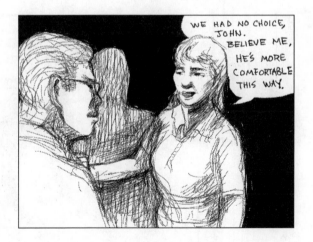

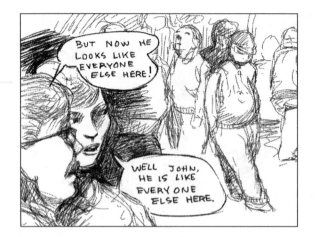

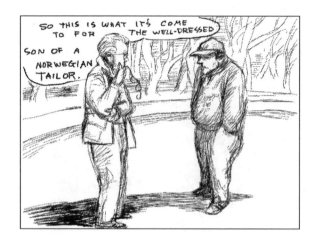

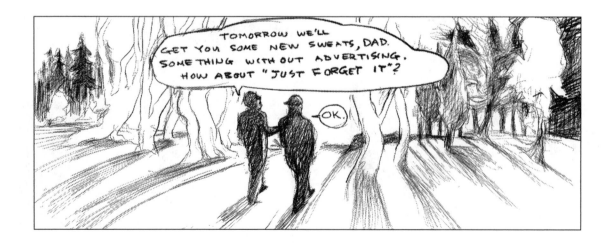

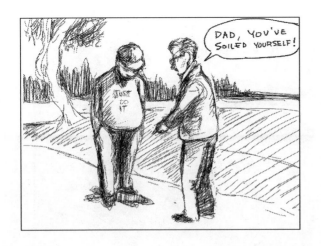

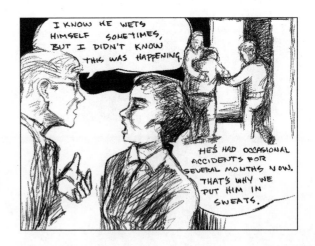

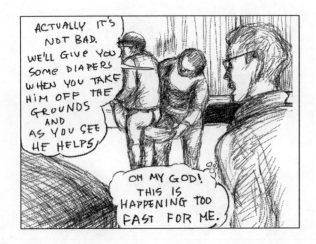

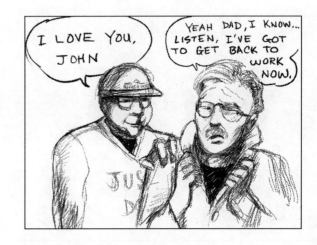

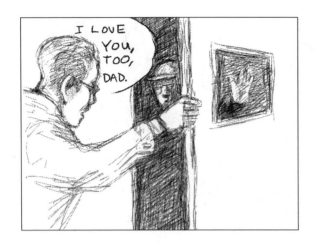

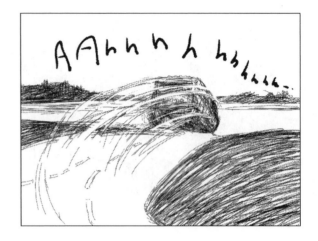

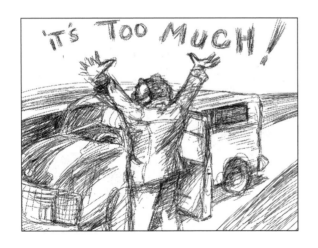

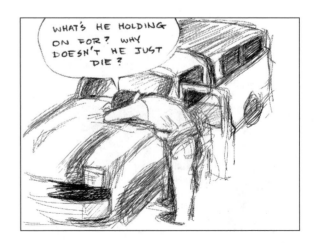

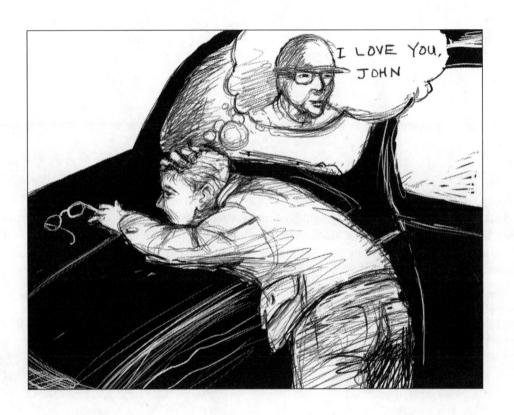

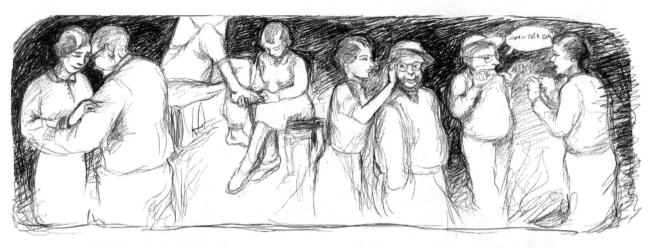

My sister Ruth returned again from the Middle East and settled in Portland. She slipped quickly and easily into looking after Dad's physical needs. This kindly attention from a vaguely familiar face was a welcome change for Dad, and, for a time, it seemed that he was getting his good humor back. I focused on his increasing confusion and the growing distance between us.

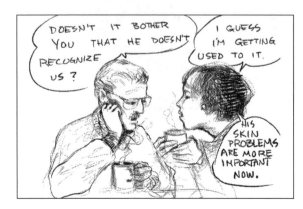

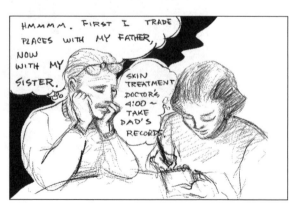

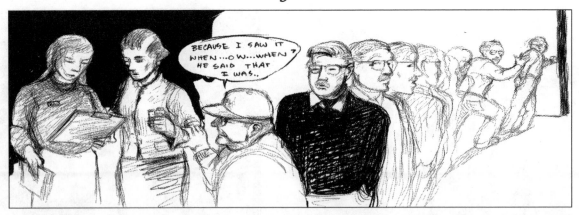

As Dad's disease progressed into the final stage and Ruth took over as care manager, I felt myself pulling away.

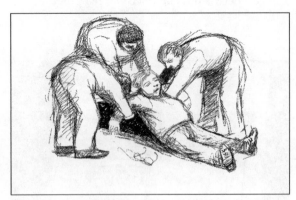

Shortly after Ruth's return, Dad fell and broke his hip. Everything changed.

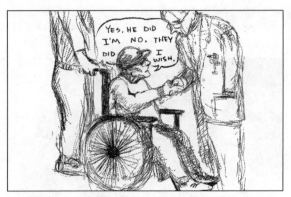

He healed quickly and returned to the nursing home in less than a week. We were assured that his physical strength would enable him to regain the use of his legs.

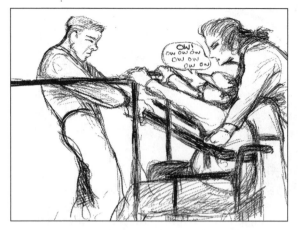

But despite all efforts, Dad never walked again.

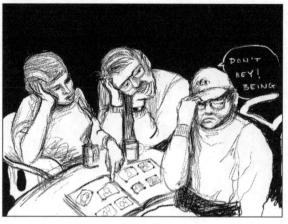

Ruth and I tried everything to engage him, but the gap between us had become too great.

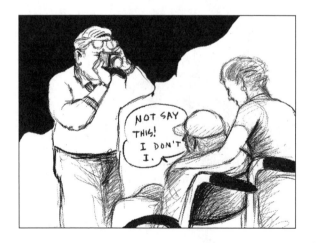

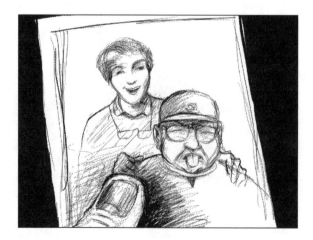

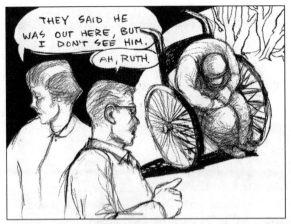

Dad's appearance changed so quickly during this time that on several occasions, Ruth and I walked right past him.

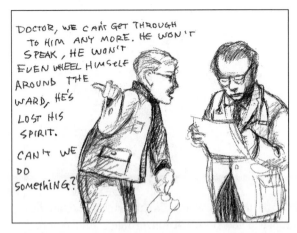

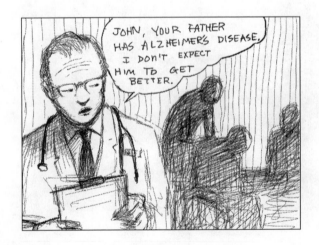

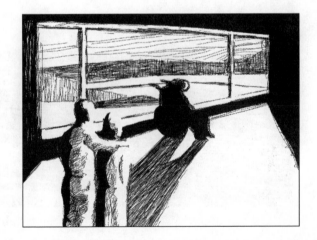

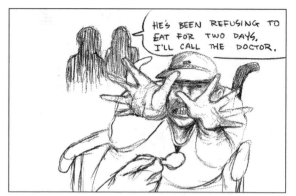

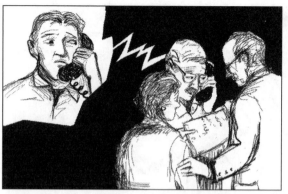

Several months after his hip surgery, Dad developed a lower intestinal problem and stopped eating. He had a similar infection years before with a long and painful recovery.

After conferring with his doctors, Ruth, Bill and I decided not to hospitalize Dad again.

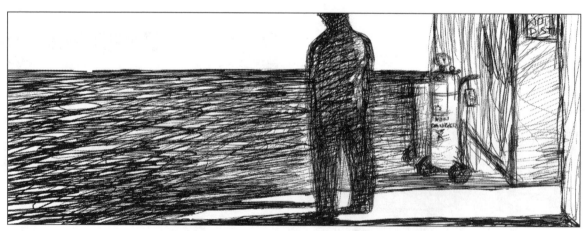

We made him as comfortable as possible and waited.

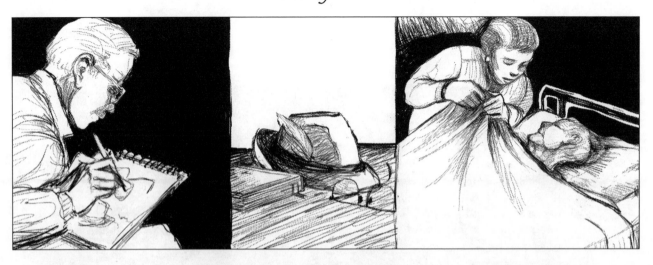

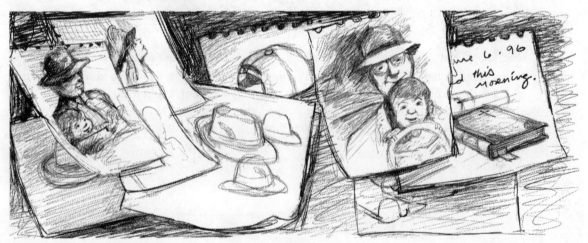

Dad died on a Sunday morning, shortly after church. He had lived in the nursing home for six years.

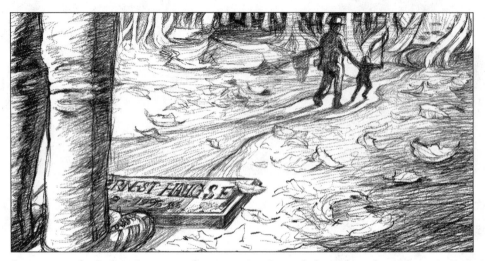

It was months before I went to the gravesite. I stood there for a long time staring at my father's name on the marker, wondering why we hadn't taken the time to shorten the distance between us when we had the chance. On the drive home, I realized, at last, I was going to miss my father.

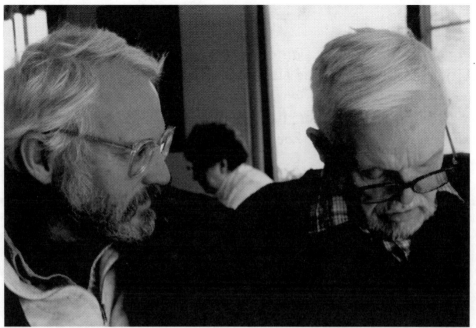

Photo by Ruth McKinney

About the Author and Artist

John Haugse received his B.A. from the San Francisco Art Institute and his M.F.A. from the University of Oregon. John has alternated professions as a painter, animator and film instructor over his thirty-year career. He has achieved honors in all three professions, including an invitation to teach animation at Harvard's Carpenter Center, a Guggenheim Award for his personal filmmaking, a

PBS airing of his film *Honore Daumier: Witness to a Century* and one-man painting exhibitions in California and Oregon.

John has just finished a film for the Dayton Museum of Natural History and is currently working on plans for an animated film of *Heavy Snow*. He lives in Portland, Oregon, with his dog, Zoe.